Use It or
Lose It!

Use It or
Lose It!

How to Keep Your Brain Fit as It Ages

Second Edition
Updated and Expanded

Allen D. Bragdon

and

David Gamon, Ph.D.

Walker & Company New York

First published in the United States of America by Allen D. Bragdon Publishers, Inc. BRAINWAVES® is a registered trademark of Allen D. Bragdon Publishers, Inc. This revised edition published in 2003 by Walker Publishing Company, Inc.

Published simultaneously in Canada by Fitzhenry and Whiteside, Markham, Ontario L3R 4T8

For information about permission to reproduce selections from this book, write to Permissions, Walker & Company, 104 Fifth Avenue, New York, New York 10011

The information in this book is intended to provide insight into how the brain functions. It is not intended for neurodiagnosis which must be conducted by qualified practitioners.

SCIENCE CONSULTANT: Suzanne Corkin, Ph.D., Professor of Behavioral Neuroscience, Department of Brain and Cognitive Sciences, Massachusetts Institute of Technology, Cambridge, MA

TECHNICAL EDITORS: Amanda Parker Ph.D., School of Psychology, University of Nottingham, United Kingdom

Book design by Carolyn Zellers.
Illustrations by Malcolm Wells and Joan Harvey Carter.

Some images reproduced with permission of LifeArt Collection Images, copyright © 1989-99 TechPOOL Studios, Cleveland, OH; Puzzle graphics copyright © 2003 by Allen D. Bragdon Publishers, Inc.

Library of Congress Cataloging-in-Publication Data
Bragdon, Allen D.
Use it or lose it! : how to keep your brain fit as it ages / by Allen D. Bragdon and David Gamon. — 2nd ed., updated and expanded.
p. cm. — (Brainwaves books)
Includes bibliographical references and index.
ISBN 0-8027-7682-5 (pbk. : alk. paper)
1. Cognition in old age. I. Gamon, David. II. Title. III. Series.
BF724.85.C64B73 2004
155.67'13 — dc22 2003062167

Visit Walker & Company's Web site at www.walkerbooks.com

Printed in Canada

2 4 6 8 10 9 7 5 3 1

Contents

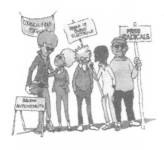

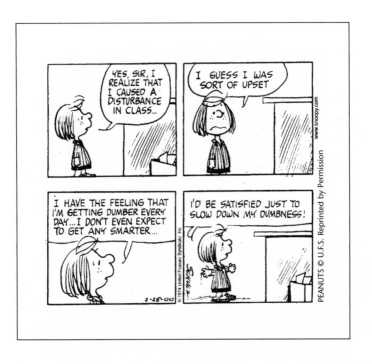

Introduction

If you play with it, your mind will grow

The central goal of this book is to explain in plain language the most current information about what impacts brain health and provide practical tools to help make sure that impact will be beneficial rather than detrimental.

Section 1 explains, in nontechnical language, the most recent, crucial research on humans that points to the role of mental, physical, and social stimulation in maintaining brain function. As it goes, it spells out practical things you can do every day to help your brain stay healthy so you can compete professionally, improve the quality of your life as a senior and lower the risk of Alzheimer's. Like walking or jogging, they cost nothing, are nontaxable and fat free.

Section 2 offers information to help recognize signs of brain failure, how to evaluate how you are doing, and gives you tests to measure your mental performance skills against norms at various ages. There you will also find the latest research results on substances and environmental conditions that can harm the brain.

Section 3 translates current findings in the neurosciences that have practical applications to everyday life. Though it does not require any technical knowledge at all it provides information in more depth for those who want to know what has been discovered regarding outmoded beliefs, new findings, and some practical ways to apply them to improve cognitive performance in real life situations.

Section 4 is fun. Research with laboratory animals long ago showed that increasing mental activity by constantly changing the playthings in some of the mouse cages to challenge the animals in them to investigate and explore also increased the size and quality of their brain cells. Recent research confirms that forcing the mind to investigate and explore unfamiliar stimuli improves performance in adult human brains.

The appendix offers the lowdown on Alzheimer's disease (AD) informed by current research results. It includes easily administered tests used in preliminary diagnosis of AD and other crippling brain failures. Technical references listed at the end of each section and arranged by subject, along with the index, enable the reader who is interested in a specific aspect of brain function to easily locate where to find it and learn more about it.

But how to do this while balancing work, family and physical exercise? Here is help. We have assembled 36 mental conditioning exercises designed to sharpen the six mental skill-sets that you use to get through your day. These mental pushups are presented as entertaining puzzles at various levels of difficulty, with optional hints to help readers get started without having to give up. Try one every morning like a crossword puzzle to wake up peak-performance circuits in the brain that may normally not be used.

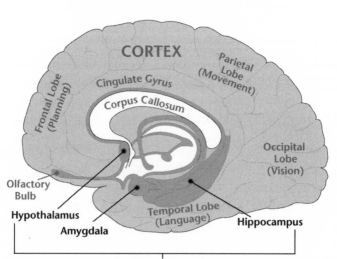

CORTEX

Parietal Lobe (Movement)

Frontal Lobe (Planning)

Cingulate Gyrus

Corpus Callosum

Occipital Lobe (Vision)

Olfactory Bulb

Hypothalamus

Amygdala

Temporal Lobe (Language)

Hippocampus

LIMBIC SYSTEM

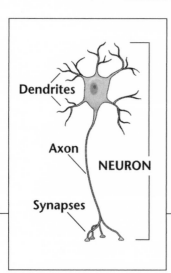

Dendrites

Axon

NEURON

Synapses

The diagram above shows the brain's interior with the "gray matter" of the thinking cortex atop the more primitive limbic system, which controls instinctive responses, emotions, and memory.

At left, a diagram of a common type of brain cell. Electro-chemical impulses travel down the axon through the synapses to the dendrites of adjacent cells This causes them to fire impulses to other cells.

MENTAL LAPSES THAT YOU *DON'T* NEED TO WORRY ABOUT

SIGNS OF NORMAL, HEALTHY AGE-RELATED DECLINE

RESEARCH PROVES THAT "USING IT PRESERVES IT"

MAKING YOUR MEMORY WORK FOR YOU

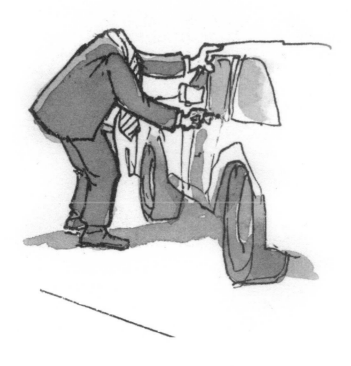

Signs of Normal, Healthy Age-Related Decline

All the mental changes described in this section can be grouped under the quaint-sounding umbrella of "benign senescent forgetfulness" — things that may be inconvenient or embarrassing, perhaps, but not in themselves dangerous or a sign of a less benign forgetfulness to come. Alzheimer's is certainly deserving of some of the dread it evokes, but even at age 80, the chances of memory lapses being benign are a lot better than the chances of having dementia, by a ratio of about 4 to 1. Even so, the fact that even healthy aging is accompanied by changes in the same brain regions that are damaged by Alzheimer's is usually far from reassuring. That means that older people who never develop Alzheimer's may experience changes in mental abilities that look like early dementia but are not.

Driving the brain

Who pays the highest premium for car insurance? You probably know the answer: teenage boys. Statistics show that young males have the highest accident rates and are the worst drivers on the roads.

Why? Although reaction time, alertness, concentration, and other skills that are crucial for safe driving are at their peak early in life, teenage boys crave excitement, enjoy taking risks, and do not concern themselves with consequences. With age and experience, good judgment and wisdom develop, and these characteristics are more important for safe driving than the swiftness of youth.

Driving is a good analogy for mental abilities such as memory, learning, and concentration. With the aging brain, as with the mature body, reaction time slows. On timed tests involving mental skills, older people generally perform more poorly than younger individuals. The same physical changes that result in slower reflexes may also make it harder to remember names, follow two conversations at once, or remember the details of a recent movie. However, the good news is that cognitive skill is similar to driving skill: Even though reaction time slows, performance can be maintained — even improved — by practicing, using brain circuits, and keeping them busy.

Good low down on brain slow-down
Starting in the second decade of life, brain cells and their connections to other cells lose power and some cells are even lost if not used regularly. This slow-down in mental processing causes an older person to take longer to arrive at a solution to a problem. However, don't despair. The end solution may be just as "correct" as the one arrived at quickly by a younger individual.

Here's an example. In a recent experiment, researchers presented young and old subjects with awkward scenarios depicting real-life problems. For example, one scenario involved a young man who stomps into his landlord's office complaining about new neighbors in an apartment directly above his. They have several dogs that keep him up all night with their frolicking and barking. The subjects were given two minutes to think of as many solutions as possible. Only solutions judged reasonable ("Attempt to negotiate a solution with the neighbor") counted; unreasonable ones ("Kill the dogs") did not. Older subjects came up with significantly fewer solutions in the allotted time than younger subjects, but their solutions were judged to be higher quality on average. Ultimately, there was no difference between young and old subjects in the number of good solutions they proposed.

Why can't I remember like I used to?

Older individuals tend to perform worse on memory-related tasks even when they are not under time constraints. For example, after leisurely reading a daily newspaper or magazine article, an 80-year-old will likely have more trouble remembering the details than a 20-year-old will. Why? A reduction in processing speed may be the reason. Since new information is processed more slowly as one ages, researchers think memory traces of one piece of information may start to disappear before the next piece of information is received and laid down. The aging brain may not efficiently "reach back" and combine the pieces into a meaningful, coherent whole, essential for remembering the details.

Is mental deterioration "normal?"

A certain degree of mental slowing is inevitable with age, but the amount of decrease in mental processing

A Skill That Does Not Decline with Age: Vocabulary

Every one of these adjectives relates to an animal. Which animal? (They get harder farther down the list.)

1. feline	6. piscine
2. canine	7. lupine
3. equine	8. bovine
4. leonine	9. aquiline
5. porcine	10. phocine

(Hint: In Nabokov's novel *Lolita,* the narrator Humbert refers to Lolita's mother, lounging by the swimming pool in a black one-piece, as "her *phocine* mama."

Scoring:
    5 = average   6 = good   7 = very good
    8 = excellent   9-10 = outstanding

speed and the results of such slowing are not set in stone. For instance, there is enormous variability in the "normal" or "acceptable" age-related changes in people who do not develop Alzheimer's. Individuals differ dramatically. Some 80-year-olds show obvious deterioration in mental agility even though they are physically healthy, while others who are quite physically ill show little mental change at all.

So should we really accept the "acceptable" changes? We need to ask why some people change more than others and to ask ourselves if anything can be done about it. Later on in this section, we will discuss some interesting research that indicates some "normal" signs of aging can be prevented by exercising the mind in a certain way. See the appendix for a list of behaviors that identify normal age-related decline in processing speed compared with behaviors that point to advanced dementia and Alzheimer's.

Why does it get harder to think of the right word?
There's a joke that goes like this. Older people are faced with a dilemma: they know more words, but they can't remember them! Vocabulary improves with age. What declines is the kind of mental nimbleness needed to access all those words on the fly. Everybody knows exactly what this feels like: you know the word, it may even be on the tip of your tongue, but you can't quite think of it. So you fumble around, hem and haw, and hope the word pops into your mind while you stall for time. Maybe it does, or maybe it doesn't and you have to move on, feeling like a bit of a fool. Of course, you'll soon think of the word, two minutes too late to do you any good.

Why multiple-choice questions are easier than fill-in-the-blank
Why does this happen? The knowledge of the meaning of a word and the ability to think of the right word under time pressure are two different abilities handled by different brain systems. Thinking quickly of the *mot juste* — the act that psychologists call lexical access — relies on exactly the kind of frontal-lobe brain activity that tends to get a little sluggish for everybody, even for those who never develop Alzheimer's. That difference between *knowing* (recognition) and *using* (recall) a word is why exam questions using fill-in-the-blanks demand

Some Age-related Memory Changes Can Be Corrected by Using the Right Strategy

When encouraged to apply the right strategy, older brains switch on the relevant memory circuits as effectively as younger brains. But older brains will still create "noise" by activating brain regions irrelevant to successful memorization. Even if they can't completely undo the effects of age, memorization strategies can help an older brain regain a more youthful learning curve.

#1: A young brain activating the left frontal region associated with successful memorization

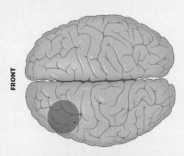

#2: An old brain underactivating that left region while overactivating an irrelevant region on the right side

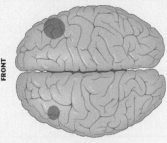

#3: An old brain successfully activating the left region when encouraged to perform a "deep" encoding task, but still activating the irrelevant right-hemisphere region

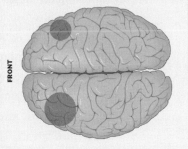

more mental effort than multiple-choice no matter how young or old you are. But that difference naturally grows larger as you grow older.

Modern brain-imaging technology has allowed researchers to observe young and old brains in the process of successfully memorizing or recalling something. They can now identify precise locations in the brain that are activated when those memory processes are working effectively and efficiently (see page 7).

If older subjects are simply told to memorize something or retrieve information from memory, the prefrontal memory regions are *underactivated* relative to younger brains, and relative to brains that are successfully memorizing or remembering. Also, as older brains desperately attempt to tap networks that are actually irrelevant to the task at hand, activity in their prefrontal area looks more scattered than younger brains.

A good memory uses a good strategy for remembering
The good news is that older brains will activate the proper regions just as effectively as younger brains as long as they're prompted to use the right strategy. If older subjects are told to remember a list of words, they tend to do a worse job than younger subjects. But they perform equally as well if the researchers suggest an effective strategy, say to think about the meanings of the words by judging, for example, whether each word represents a concrete or abstract entity. Both groups then activate the exact regions associated with successful memorization. The mental resources are still there as brains age but they're not accessed as automatically.

Older people have to, in effect, put more effort into making an effort. For them, those frontal systems still work, they just need a little extra push.

How to use this information to improve memory?
First, don't panic if you're having a harder time remembering the right word at the right time. It doesn't mean there's something wrong with your brain, nor does it mean you have Alzheimer's. Second, *expect* to have to put out a little extra effort to recall something by picturing it in your mind or pausing to relate it to something you already know. Third, you most likely have more words to search through than you did when you were a teenager. That should be a source of pride. A fall-off in your brain's efficiency in thinking of a word is better than not knowing that word at all, don't you think?

There's more good news. Even though your brain is probably not going to regain the processing speed it had when you were 20, many frontal-lobe skills can be improved through practice. That means you can compensate for slower processing speed by developing new techniques to aid recall. Storing data into memory came automatically to you when you were younger. Now putting the effort into smart strategies and exercising those frontal brain circuits can keep them working well. The cells are healthy. They just tend to "nod off" when you need them.

Where the brain remembers
The kinds of memory loss that happen as we age can be understood in terms of changes in certain structures in the brain. Two areas in the brain that decline in even

healthy older people are the hippocampus and the frontal lobes. The hippocampus is a structure within the brain that plays a crucial role in processing incoming information and creating long-term memories out of them, and (to varying degrees) in retrieving memories from storage sites scattered widely throughout the cortex. The frontal lobes play a role in devising strategies for organizing and memorizing new information, in effortful attempts to retrieve that information from memory, and in remembering the source of the information.

Recalling the original source of something you "know" is hard

This is called *source memory*. A failure in source memory reveals itself whenever we recall something that someone told us without remembering who it was who told us, or when, or where, or why. This is a particular problem for children, whose frontal lobes have not yet developed fully, as well as for older adults, whose frontal lobes may have lost some of their mass. Frontal-lobe-based memory failure may also show itself as a tendency to forget to follow through on plans — a problem, once again, common to young children and older adults alike. All these changes are considered normal, and they are not a sign of dementia.

The brain networks that develop most slowly in childhood are also the first to decline in adulthood; the frontal lobes especially.

Mild, but sometimes embarrassing, lapses that are normal

An overall increase in the time needed to figure things out or to solve problems is normal. It is also typical for older people to have a harder time keeping something in their mind — say, a telephone number — long enough to perform some task with it — say, dial it. It also gets harder to organize information efficiently, to sort out the relevant from the irrelevant, and to keep the memory of one piece of information from interfering with another. Most, if not all, of these skills center on the brain's frontal lobes. The frontal lobes house skills that tend to be complex and effortful, and that need to be practiced both in school and years afterward to keep them sharp. Frontal-lobe skills are unique to humans. They are the opposite of "hardwired" instincts. That is why they require *conscious effort* to do their thing.

It makes a notable difference when older people get into the habit of making an effort to focus hard on a task and develop problem-solving strategies. In fact, older people have an advantage because they have more knowledge networks behind the frontal lobes to help them understand, learn, and remember things. They can organize new information so that it's firmly embedded in knowledge already acquired. Then, the mental effort of prodding the frontal lobes into action is no longer as necessary when it comes time to access that knowledge.

Injuries to the front part of the brain have long provided evidence that the frontal lobes are responsible for helping people lead a productive life and solve problems in a rational manner. They marshal and organize skills handled by other parts of the brain. Those are abilities that psychologists refer to as "executive" skills. You might think of the frontal cortex as the location of

Memory Span Test

An important skill required for effective working memory is the ability to store information temporarily and then refer back to it on demand. This test demonstrates that ability.

(1) Read the following sentence aloud, then turn to page 14 and answer the question printed in the left margin.

"The bus driver motioned the red truck to continue, which turned left, stopped by the third driveway, and sounded its horn twice."

(2) Read the following sentence. Then try to answer the questions in the right margin of page 15:

"The acrobat discussed game theory with a trained harbor seal riding on a tiger in a wagon pulled by a white stallion."

the brain's supervisory system, a system that orchestrates the efforts of the workers on the factory floor.

When people age they find it increasingly difficult to harness and direct their brain's ability to achieve goals and solve problems. It isn't so much a matter of *having* the skills as *using* them effectively.

"Working" memory is the executive's best tool

A short-term memory system known as *working memory* (WM) is the ability to keep information in mind while the brain manipulates it in some way, a task that commonly becomes more difficult with aging. For example, to multiply 7 X 13 in your head, your brain must remember the numbers involved — 7 and 13 — and then perform an operation on them (multiplication). To do that, you might break the problem down into 7

X 10, plus 7 X 3. Then, your brain must remember
what it has accomplished at each step, as it proceeds to
further steps. This combination of short-term memory
and on-line monitoring and manipulation is a demon-
stration of WM at work.

A computer test of working memory

Psychologists test WM skill with a grid of designs like
that shown here. The subject is seated in front of a
computer screen with this
series of designs on it and is
told to point to any one of
the designs in the grid. As
soon as he does this, a different screen appears with all
the same designs arranged in
a different pattern. Now, he
has to point to any one of
the designs except the one he
already pointed to on the
first screen. And so it contin-

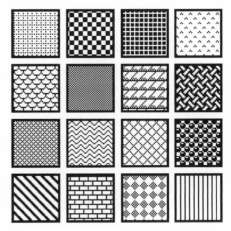

ues, with the designs appearing in a different configura-
tion each time, and the subject's task always being to
point to any one that he had not already pointed to
before.

This task is difficult because it places a burden on short-
term memory while also challenging executive skills.
Short-term memory must retain every pattern that has
been selected, then identify one that has not been
selected before by pointing to it. Obviously, part of the
brain's task is to devise strategies that will minimize the
chance of making an error.

From page 12, #1: What direction did the truck turn?

People whose frontal brain lobes have been injured have a particularly hard time on tests like this. Older people also perform worse than average on tests of executive skills, which suggests that those are skills that tend to deteriorate with age. There are several theories about exactly what changes take place in a healthy older brain to give rise to those changes in mental abilities. Certain brain regions lose some of their volume due either to a loss of connections between cells or supporting white matter cells beneath the cortex, or both.

The basic point

With normal aging, brain cells are still there even if they're functioning less efficiently. Countless studies have shown that, even in old age, neurons will change their structure in response to what their owner chooses to do with them. In particular, the connections between brain cells provided by dendrites and axons can be increased or decreased depending on whether or not they're used. Not only that, but your brain creates *brand-new* neurons for use in some of the same brain regions that tend to shrink with age. But — here's the catch — you have to use those neurons as your brain creates them if you want your brain to retain them. Only then can you be reasonably sure that they'll be there the next time you need them.

Can you know too much?

As a matter of fact the accumulation of experiences amassed since childhood can get in the way of using your brain to accommodate new experiences. Your brain can't "fill up" with information. Its capacity to learn and remember is unlimited. However, the more experiences you've had, the easier it is to get them confused. Memory researchers have recognized for a long time that one reason for apparent memory failures is having too much material to work with. How exactly?

From page 12, #2:
What theory did the seal discuss? What were the last words of the two sentences on page 12?

It is hard to remember a lot of unorganized data dumped on you all at once. There are limits to what the brain can memorize by rote repetition. Unless you spend a very long time repeating and rehearsing random data over and over in many sessions it will be lost. Again, the way to transfer bits of new information into long-term memory is to organize them in a way that makes it meaningful by associating each bit with something already available for recall.

New information or experiences tend to "overwrite" less recent ones

Another way too much information can get in the way of memory is called *memory interference*. Here's an example from Harvard memory researcher Daniel Schacter: *I can remember what I had for breakfast today, but not what I had for breakfast on this day a year ago, because I have had many breakfasts since then that interfere with my ability to pick out any single one from the crowd.*

You may have noticed that if you read two short stories in one sitting, the second will make it harder to remember the first after you've finished reading both. Interference can work the other way, too. If your friend changes his/her phone number, it may take a while before the old one stops getting in the way of memorizing the new one.

What did I come into this room to get?

It happens to everybody. You think of something that needs attention in another room. On the way, something else comes to mind or you step on the cat. Soon you'll be standing in the next room wondering what it is that you went there to do.

The trick to preventing that kind of memory lapse is to make an effort to focus on whatever task it is you're off to perform and keep any distractions at bay until you're done. (If you do that and still forget within a few seconds what you were supposed to be doing, then you'd have reason to worry.) The trouble is, if you add up all the little things you could potentially focus on every second of every day, there are far too many. So you put your mind on autopilot, and for most things that works just fine.

Are lapses like these that interfere with memory the harbinger of dementia? Not at all. Just as source memory confusion happens more frequently as you get older, interference becomes more of a problem as well. You must continually force your brain to keep things straight as easily as it used to. An older brain can't operate on autopilot as it used to without confusion about what you did, what you're going to do, and exactly what it was that somebody told you.

Divided attention; multi-tasking and focus
Keeping your mind focused on a task is hard work. That's one reason it's easier to do one thing at a time than to try to do a lot of things simultaneously. At any age, there are limits to attentional capacity. The brain can't concentrate on one thing forever or tune out all distractions or pay attention to everything at once.

Attentional capacity is a lot like the electrical system in a house. As long as too many appliances are not running at once, everything works just fine. When too many are drawing from limited juice the circuit breaks. And the older the house, the smaller the load it is wired for.

Doing any one thing that demands focused concentration taxes brain capacity; two things simultaneously is *much* harder especially if both things depend on the same brain system, It's easy to hum while you read, or have a conversation while you eat, but a lot harder to have a conversation while you read. Reading and talking use the same brain circuits; reading and humming do not.

As with working memory, mental quickness, and executive skills, scientists have simple tests that confirm what common sense tells you about age-related changes in your ability to do several things at once. The technical term for what they test is *divided attention*, a skill that psychologists test by getting subjects to wear headphones with, say, one stream of words coming into the left ear and a different one coming into the right. The task then is to repeat back the words that you heard in your two different ears, in order, without jumbling up left with right. Older people do worse on divided attention tests than younger people do.

Fatigue interferes with concentration ability
If you're tired, it's more difficult to tune out distractions. And as with other frontal-lobe skills, mental multitasking gets harder with age. In real life outside the psychology lab, that shows itself in greater difficulty following a conversation when a lot of other people in

the room are talking, or a tendency to miss the correct freeway off-ramp while someone in the car is haranguing you about your choice of radio station.

Why is Alzheimer's a disease while normal aging is "healthy" if the same parts of the brain are impacted by both?

Perhaps the most important difference is that Alzheimer's destroys brain cells that are needed for proper memory function and mental control. Medical doctors used to believe that brain cell death was a natural part of normal aging, a view suggested by evidence of a shrinkage in older brains, especially in the frontal lobes and hippocampus. But it now looks more likely that the changes in an aging Alzheimer's-free brain are a matter of a drop in the quality of brain cells rather than their quantity. In other words, individual brain cells don't die, but they may become smaller and less effective by losing some of their branches that let them communicate with other brain cells.

Shrinking gray and white cells

Beneath the gray matter of the brain's "thinking cap," so-called "white matter" may shrink as well. White matter consists of long branches called *axons* that serve as long-distance connections between neurons in different parts of the brain. Loss of white matter volume may be due to a loss of *myelin*, the white-colored insulation wrapped around the axon that allows it to carry nerve impulses quickly and efficiently.

On a cellular level, a shrinkage of gray matter cells and a loss in nerve transmission speed due to thinning of the white matter's myelin may underlie all of the "normal," healthy age-related changes discussed in this section. Both changes are obvious possible causes of the slowing of response time and the loss of efficiency typical in an aging brain.

A few of these changes in a brain as it ages still appear to be unavoidable. A fall-off in processing speed may be just as inevitable as a slowing of reaction time with physical skills. The best way to respond to changes like that is to compensate for them by adjusting behavior. Some examples, if you talk on a cell phone while driving at age 80, you run a greater risk of having an accident than you would at age 40. Activities and hobbies that rely on pure mental quickness may naturally become less enjoyable, too. And the "noise factor" may become more important when considering where to go out to dinner.

The fundamental difference between disease and aging

But there are other ways to compensate for a changing brain by adjusting how you *use* mental resources, rather than just passively accepting those changes as natural. Most research shows that, for many of the differences between younger and older people, the changes lie in how *automatically* and *effortlessly* certain brain-based faculties kick into gear as they're needed. That's very different from not having those faculties at all, and therein lies the fundamental difference between healthy aging and Alzheimer's. An older person must put conscious effort into doing things that used to come effortlessly, and alter strategies for cementing new experiences into recallable memory, but the job can get done with a little effort — old brain or not. The kinds of skills that tend to weaken with age must be used and practiced at every age to be maintained. How you use your brain feeds back on your brain's structure, which in turn affects your abilities. That spiral can go up or down, depending on the choices you make. Some of the most intriguing recent research suggests you can take steps to mitigate many of those age-related changes that are considered normal. While those things won't help to cure Alzheimer's once you have it, some studies point to ways you can use your brain that might help you to *avoid* Alzheimer's. For those, read on.

RESEARCH PROVES THAT "USING IT PRESERVES IT"

There is compelling evidence that problem-solving and memory skills do not have to get worse with age, even though they may require more effort to keep them working well. One source of evidence that not all kinds of "normal" mental slowdown are inevitable comes from people who continue to challenge their minds into old age. Here's an example.

A few years ago, psychologists at the University of California, Berkeley, decided to test the assumption that typical age-related cognitive changes necessarily come with the territory of aging. Their findings suggest that some of those changes are not inevitable, and that working memory and executive skills may be maintained by the degree to which people challenge themselves mentally as they age.

The study tested the cognitive skills of five groups of people: one group of young people and one group of old people from a variety of professions, and younger, middle-aged, and older professors at Berkeley. The mental abilities tested were reaction time, working memory, prose recall, and something called Paired Associate

SELF-TEST: Paired Associate Learning
A Skill That Declines with Age, No Matter How Sharp
You Keep Your Mind

Paired associate learning means the memorization of arbitrary pairs (faces, names, and so forth). Healthy older people naturally perform worse on this kind of task than their younger counterparts, even if they have kept themselves mentally fit. The problem with paired associate learning is that the pairs are arbitrary and do not fit into any kind of pre-existing knowledge base. In order to memorize the pairs, you have to apply some sort of mnemonic trick or other, a frontal-lobe-based technique that apparently comes less automatically to you as you get older.

You will need a timer. Your task is to remember which female face goes with which male face. Study the six pairs of faces on this page for four seconds each (twenty-four seconds total) and then continue to the instructions below.

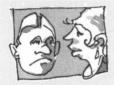 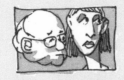 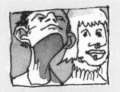

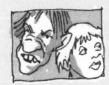 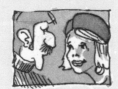 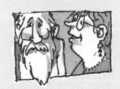

Next, look at the box of six male faces on page 24. Match each male face to one of the female faces in the box below, following the pairings on this page to the best of your recollection. Do not spend longer than a minute. (On these quick timed tasks, ask a friend to time you so you are not preoccupied with the stopwatch.) Repeat the task twice, observing the same time limits.

Learning, which is the memorization of arbitrary pairs, such as names and faces (see Self-test, page 22). The nonprofessors showed the typical age-related decline in all these cognitive skills — that is, the younger ones performed significantly better than the older ones. So far, no surprises.

Where the older professors held their own
Among the professors, however, the pattern of results was different. The older professors (ages 60-71) did show the typical declines in reaction time and paired associate learning compared to middle-aged (45-59) and younger (30-44) professors. In that way, they were just like other people.

But on other tests the older professors' performance was more interesting. In the last section, we described a test that psychologists use to measure working memory and executive skills

Essentially, this task was designed to trigger *proactive* interference: earlier-remembered selections interfere with the ability to remember or keep track of choices made in the second trial. Since, normally, interference afflicts older people more, the group of older non-professors did indeed show the typical age-related vulnerability to proactive interference, performing worse in the second trial than the first. The older professors, on the other hand, made *fewer* mistakes in the second trial. In other words, they showed none of the normal age-related interference problems.

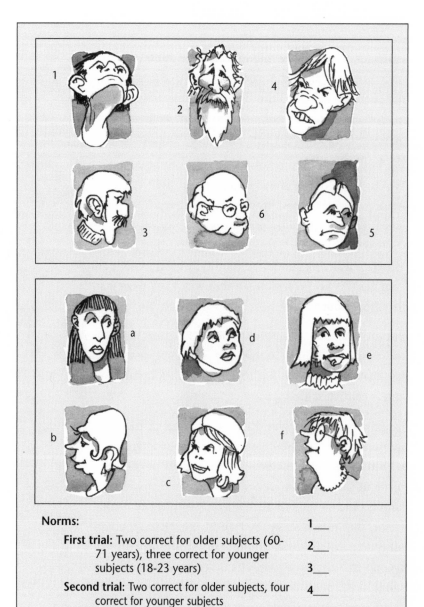

Norms:

> **First trial:** Two correct for older subjects (60-71 years), three correct for younger subjects (18-23 years)
>
> **Second trial:** Two correct for older subjects, four correct for younger subjects
>
> **Third trial:** Three correct for older subjects, five correct for younger subjects

1___
2___
3___
4___
5___
6___

The same pattern arose in the prose recall test. In the general population, older people do worse than younger people when they have to remember details from a passage that has just been read to them. Among the professors, on the other hand, there were no age differences in performance. Older professors did just as well as, or even better than, younger ones.

These findings suggest that people don't have to accept all of the kinds of cognitive loss considered "inevitable" as they age. In their work and intellectual interests, the older professors sustained a high level of activity in grappling with conceptually challenging material on a daily basis. It may be, then, that the daily practice these senior professors had in acquiring and organizing new knowledge helped them to perform well on these tasks.

Where the older professors faltered

As mentioned above, there were tests of reaction time and paired associate learning on which the professors' tests that showed poorer performance with increased age help to reveal a pattern that provides insight into the changes that are inevitable with age and those that are not. Why would intellectual exercise not have a protective effect against poorer performance in tests of reaction time and paired associate learning?

As the authors of the study pointed out, an obvious answer is that reaction time and paired associate learning abilities have little to do with conceptual skills that professors use on a daily basis. Many of the tests psychologists use to evaluate the memory skills of all kinds of people seem divorced from real life. Simply memo-

Trail Making Test

The Trail Making Test is a test of complex visual scanning, attention, mental flexibility, and motor speed. It can be used to help verify head trauma or dementia, but even among normal, healthy people performance on the test tends to decline dramatically with age. This is a timed test, so you will need a clock, watch, or stopwatch.

Instructions: On the opposite page are some letters and numbers. Begin at letter A ("start") and draw a line from A to 1, 1 to B, B to 2 and so on, in order until you reach the last number ("end"). Note the time taken to complete the entire series.

Norms: The time taken to complete this test varies with age as well as with education level. For example, the average healthy 15-to-20-year-old needs 47 seconds to finish the trail, while the average healthy 70-to-79-year-old needs 180 seconds. Normal adults 40-60 years old with less than 12 years of education need 102 seconds, while those with at least 16 years of education need a little less than one minute. The following table shows the norms by age group. You can see how large the range is even among healthy, non-demented adults.

Trail Making Test: Time in Seconds Needed by Healthy Subjects to Complete, by Age

Percentile	15-20	20-39	40-49	50-59	60-69	70-79
90	26	45	30	55	62	79
75	37	55	52	71	83	122
50	47	65	78	80	95	180
25	59	85	102	128	142	210
10	70	98	126	162	174	350

(Note: A score in the 90th percentile means 90 percent of people in that age group score lower, etc.)

(Source: U.S. Army Individual Test Battery)

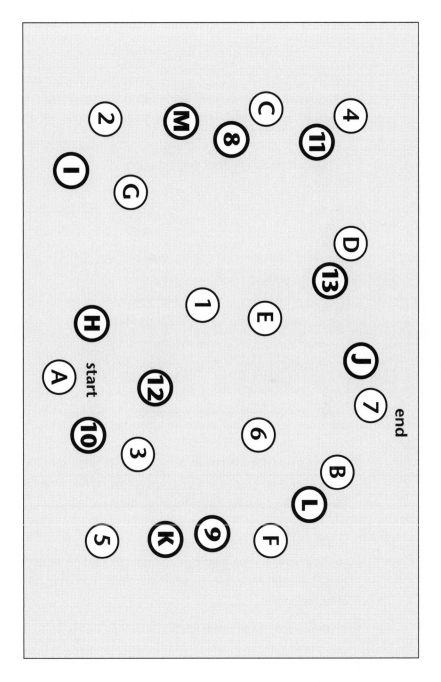

Recognition vs. Recollection List #1

Take a minute to memorize the items on this shopping list. Then cover the list and write down as many items as you can recall. Next, turn the page and look at List #2 there. It contains some of the items listed below. Which ones? Which was easier? Moral: Recognition is easier than recollection, especially when you get older.

Milk	Tomatoes
Eggs	Soup
Lettuce	Carrots
Onions	Swiss cheese
Mayonnaise	Yogurt
Ice cream	Apples
Green beans	Peanut Butter
Ham	Margarine
Ketchup	Ground beef
Salt	Broccoli

rizing associations between pairs of names, for example, or memorizing a list of name-face pairs, has little to do with how people normally integrate new information with pre-existing knowledge. This conclusion also applies to other standard tests of short-term memory, such as memorizing a string of randomly chosen numbers. Reaction time, too, has little to do with conceptual knowledge.

Older people generally have a harder time with high-level planning, organizing, and problem-solving skills than do younger people. These quintessentially human executive skills are housed in the brain's frontal lobes, which tend to slow down with age. So the daily intellectual exercise of the older professors may either have had a protective effect against frontal-lobe deterioration, or given them strategies to overcome this deterioration, just as an older baseball player can develop strategies to compensate for slower reflexes.

The encouraging thing about studies like this is that they suggest that for some of the more important cognitive skills — higher-level conceptual skills as opposed to mere reaction time or arbitrary memorization — performance can be maintained at youthful levels if the effort is made to do so. This makes sense in the light of other studies that have shown that intellectually stimulating activities practiced on a regular basis may reduce the risk of Alzheimer's (see Practical Ways to Apply Scientifically Proven Research, page 102).

Strategies for maintaining performance

If you want to keep up your cognitive performance, it helps to shift your strategies from ones that rely on skills that do weaken (reaction time or arbitrary memorization, for example) to ones that don't, or don't have to. It's no coincidence that some of the strategies that can help maintain memory in old age are the same ones that can make memory better at any age. In particular, when you move data from the "arbitrary" box into the "meaningful" one, you'll remember it better.

Elaborate encoding

Many of the conscious tricks people use to help them

SELF-TEST: Elaborate Encoding Strategy Trick

Look at the list of eight words below. For each word, answer this question: *How many vowels does the word have?* Do that, then continue reading.

cat chair cup rose
shirt grass ball door

Next, answer this question: *How many curved letters does the word have?* Now do that for each word, then continue reading.

Now, cover the list with your hand and repeat back as many of the words as possible. Do it, then read on.

Now, try this. For each word, ask yourself a question like this: "Is a cat a kind of animal?" "Is a chair a kind of furniture?" Do that for each of the words, then cover them again and see how many you can remember now.

---

remember rely on something known as *elaboration*, which is essentially a process of making new things meaningful.

The self-test above calls for two different memorization strategies that had nothing to do with the words' meanings, just shape and spelling. The brain finds it much easier to remember the words with the third technique that invoked the words' meaning, thus linking it with some data already in permanent memory. That technique is an illustration of the elaborative encoding strategy, which integrates the new fact into existing knowledge, thus making it more meaning-ful and memorable.

If you take the time and trouble to go through a process of elaborative encoding of something you want to remember, that will help you remember it better at any age. But there's good evidence that younger brains have less need of taking the "time and trouble" than older ones. As with so many other frontal-lobe skills, the encoding of information happens more naturally and automatically in youth.

In PET scans of a brain in action, the effort to memo-rize something like a list of words lights up the frontal lobe. Older brains show less activity in the precise "suc-cessful memorization" region, and they show more ran-

---

Recognition vs. Recollection List #2

Look at the grocery list below. It contains some of the items included in List #1 on page 28 Which ones? Which was easier?

Cream	Bread
Eggs	Soup
Lettuce	Peppers
Onions	Swiss cheese
Mustard	Yogurt
Ice cream	Apples
Spinach	Peanut Butter
Ham	Margarine
Olives	Ground beef
Salt	Broccoli

dom, scattershot activity in other parts of the brain that don't aid in the task. However, an older brain will remember a word list just as well as a younger brain as long as the older brain's owner makes a point of applying a strategy of *elaborative* encoding.

Avoiding common embarrassments: "Your name again?"

In social situations, the fact of forgetting a name can be unnerving. The fear of failing to come up with someone's name causes the brain to close down the circuits that coordinate the components of memory. Then, fear joins forces with natural mental entropy to make you draw a blank.

Just because it comes less naturally, however, does not mean it cannot be done (see Self-test, page 33). In fact, many of the conscious mnemonic tricks people use to help them remember things use an elaboration strategy. These tricks can serve to compensate when memory is not elaborating automatically and unconsciously.

Oh dear, where did I leave my car?

Someone drives to the airport to pick up a friend. The airport garage is so large it is divided up into different sections, each labeled with a letter-number combination. It will be hard to recall the arbitrary location code unless an effort is made to make it meaningful so as to encode the location in memory. For example, to convert a letter-number combination, say C-2, into something easier to remember, picture returning to the lot with the friend, who says, "I see it too" when the car is located.

SELF-TEST: How to Remember People's Names

Learning personal names is an ability that appears to vary considerably across individuals and forgetting names is the most frequent memory complaint among the elderly. Even poor name memorizers, however, can overcome this deficit through the use of simple mnemonic tricks based on an understanding that when information is encoded in a personally *meaningful* way (which is sometimes referred to as the memorization being more "elaborated"), the more likely memory is to be enhanced.

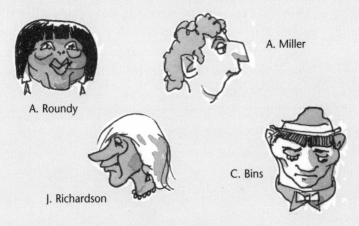

A. Miller

A. Roundy

C. Bins

J. Richardson

For each of the above face-name pairings:
1) Identify a prominent facial feature.
2) Transform the person's name into a concrete, visually vivid object.
3) Mentally picture the facial feature combined with the transformed name-object.

(Examples: A man with long hair named O'Brien; transform "O'Brien" to "lion," and visualize a lion's mane emerging from his head. A woman with heavy eyebrows named Crocker; transform "Crocker" to "cracker," and visualize a cracker on her eyebrows.) This technique can be further strengthened by performing the final step of making an *emotional* judgment of the pleasantness or unpleasantness of the image association.

Combining a random letter-number with a visual image, is a huge help. (Tip: He who writes the location code on a garage parking ticket must not leave the ticket in the car!)

A very simple trick for remembering where you left your car key, for example, might be to put it in the exact same place every time you set it down. There is nothing wrong with relying on a strategy like this and it definitely does not signal dementia.

Mnemonic tricks, or memory aids, do not strengthen the power of memory, but they do help compensate for a less-than-perfect memory. Even healthy, active 70-year-olds will need to use memory crutches if they want to memorize arbitrary details.

Making Your Memory Work for You

If you're like a lot of people, the older you get the more often you ask yourself, "Why do I forget?" Why did you forget whether or not you took your morning medicine? The name of the actor who was in that movie with the actress married to what's-his-name? Why you opened the fridge door?

"But why do I seem to forget too much these days"
You're assuming, of course, that the natural state of your brain is to remember those things, and that there's something wrong with it if it doesn't. In fact, it's just the opposite. The brain's normal state is a forgetful one. Your brain is designed to forget almost everything it encounters. That way, it won't have to waste its time thinking about the fly that crossed your field of vision at 10:32 this morning. Check out the following examples from real life.

It is amazing how much you remember automatically
We know a young professor at the peak of his cognitive power who claims he routinely forgets whether he took his pills each morning. Why? Because it's something so familiar and automatic he doesn't feel the need to pay

attention to it. Did you remember to put on your underwear this morning? To pour milk on your cereal? To open the front door *before* you stepped outside? Of course you did even though you can't remember remembering.

Why little things need the most help
Most of the routines of life are like that. The reason it's smart to always put your car keys in the same place (left pocket, purse, hall table — choose only *one*) is that little things like that are easy to forget. Your mother may worry when she forgets where she put her car keys. But, a younger person may forget where he puts his car keys all the time and not worry about it. Why? Because he always knows exactly where to find them (left pants pocket), whether or not he can remember putting them there.

Never underestimate the power of your ability to forget
Your whole life — at age 5, 15, 35 — you've been an absolute prodigy of forgetfulness and you'll remain that way until the end of your days. In fact, you've forgotten far, far more than you've ever remembered. Even the things you *think* you remember are often things you actually forgot. In addition to its power to forget, your brain comes equipped with an automatic ability to rewrite the facts of its experience. False memories are far more pervasive than you'd ever guess. Just ask two sisters about the details of a family story involving them, the cat, and Uncle Bertram's underpants in 1949.

Maybe you're asking yourself the wrong question
What you should really be asking is, "Why do I remember?" That question has many answers, but if you're

worrying about your memory the most important answer is probably this: Because you *paid attention*.

Two practical keys to paying attention that make all the difference

Trick #1: *Take mental snapshots.* Say you're on vacation in Maui, staying at a hotel right on the beach. You don't have to remember how to get to the beach, thank goodness, but you do have to remember which room you're staying in. How? Pause for a minute to take a mental snapshot of your room door viewed from the corridor. Turn around and look back the way you came to reach the room. Then, when you return to that same vantage point, you'll know which door is yours.

Trick #2: *Make mental notes.* Let's say you're in room #386. Stop and think for a minute. You're on the third floor, which is the top floor of the hotel, so the number 3 is easy. As for the 8 and the 6, 1986 was midway through Reagan's second term. Mentally noted. Or, that was the year you moved to California. Mentally noted. Or, the expression "to eighty-six" comes to mind (as in "to get rid of, do away with, or throw out"). As in what your boss will do to you if you decide to spend an extra week in Maui. Mentally noted.

These are just examples of two techniques that work anywhere, anytime. A good memory is not "automatic" all the time for anybody. The only hard part is to break down and admit that is true of you, too. Once you arm yourself with that conviction you will find that the only effort is at the beginning, when you pause to take your mental snapshot or make your mental notes. And, of course, *anyone can do this*. It makes no difference whether you think you have a "good memory" or a "bad memory." Yes, you have to put a little effort into it all day as you walk around in life, but it's not hard. It's more a matter of deciding to do it. In fact, it will become automatic after a while.

❝The one who thinks over his experiences most, and weaves them into systematic relations with each other will be the one with the best memory.❞

William James

The first step: The way memory works, paying attention consciously is most important

The brains of most other animals are hardwired to pay attention to life-supporting and life-threatening situations — and that's all. No judgment involved. Just instinct. Part of the human brain is wired that way too (a part that evolved early called the Limbic System). That is why you drop a hot fork, always remember your first kiss, or the iris in your eyes widen when you see something you want. But the human brain can also evaluate non-crisis events in terms of how they might help or harm that person in the future. The only way to remember that non-crisis event is to choose to pay attention to it consciously. This is especially critical when the situation is not routine. Remembering to do something today that you have done every day at the same time is easy, just as anything you *practice* is easy to remember. But you have to tell your brain when a *new* experience is important to you. So important that it must *pay attention* so you can use it to your benefit in the future or avoid its harm in the future.

The second step: *Linking* **new information to something you already know**

Once you have made your brain pay attention to something new you must help it *store* it.

Here is the trick: Tell your brain how the new event is similar in some ways to other data already easily recalled. Any old way will work. In fact, the weirder the better. The trick is to link the new data to established information. The more different categories of known info you can link to, the more likely your brain can find the new information when you need it again. That is why you should take a mental snapshot of what the new event looks like *and* think of something familiar that is like the new name or number *and* link it to an event from your past that is similar in some way.

Why does memory get worse as you age?

The surprising answer: *It doesn't.* Memory isn't that simple. It's not like a single muscle that you must strengthen with practice lest it atrophy with disuse. In order to understand the kinds of memory-related changes you can expect as you get older and how memory might be maintained or improved, it's important to know that memory is many skills lumped together into the word "memory."

What we loosely refer to as "memory" is, in fact, many different processes that occur in different parts of the brain. Most of us are already familiar with the basic distinction between short-term memory and long-term memory. Those are fundamentally different processes in different parts of the brain; but they are equipped to interact to create knowledge.

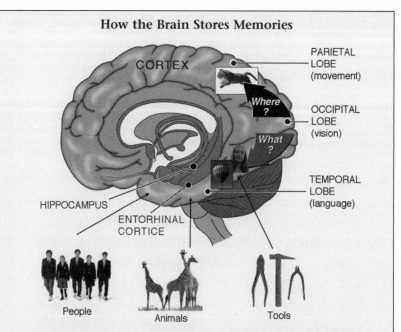

How the Brain Stores Memories

CORTEX

PARIETAL
LOBE
(movement)

Where?

OCCIPITAL
LOBE
(vision)

What?

TEMPORAL
LOBE
(language)

HIPPOCAMPUS

ENTORHINAL
CORTICE

People

Animals

Tools

Short-term memories float briefly in the neural activity of your *cortex*, the wrinkled sheet of densely packed neurons that covers the top and sides of the brain. Conversion of short- into long-term memories requires the assistance of areas in the middle of the brain (the *hippocampus* and *entorhinal cortice*). Once memories are consolidated into long-term storage, the hippocampus plays a less and less important role in retrieving them. Long-term memories are housed in many regions of the cortex, often corresponding to the parts of the brain that became activated during the initial experience of the remembered event or fact. For example, memory of sounds is stored in the Temporal Lobes near the ears; visual memories, in the Occipital area in the back. In this sense, there is no one "memory" region of the brain. The brain even stores the names of different categories of objects in different places. Faces are stored separately from foods, tools separately from animals, and animals separately from people's names.

The short and the long of memory = learning

Only a small fraction of short-term memories get converted into long-term storage. Only long-term memories literally alter your brain's structure. When the brain converts a passing piece of information into a permanent memory, it synthesizes proteins for new dendrites and axon pathways, but, first, the brain must be persuaded that the information is important enough to store. Repeating something over and over, called *rehearsal*, is one way, such as "2 times 2 is 4; 2 times 4 is 8. . . ." Sometimes a dramatic event will promote permanent storage, such as finding out that you can ride a bike without holding onto the handlebars but you crash if you take your feet off the pedals at the same time. Not much effort is needed to remember that after you pick yourself up bruised and bleeding.

Learning happens when the brain physically changes to build a new pathway

This ability to change its own physical structure in response to stimuli is called *plasticity*. Brains don't naturally lose their plasticity in old age, even though they become less *easily* malleable. One way to help maintain your brain's ability to carve new memory paths is to use it in ways that require it to change its structure on an ongoing basis — simply put, to keep learning new things. That's the "use it or lose it" principle in a nutshell. The trick to remembering something new is to relate it in some way to a fact you already know. Therefore, the more you learn, the more bits of permanent knowledge you have available to link a new fact to.

A test that proves that practice cannot increase the power of basic brain functions

The *digit span test* measures the short-term memory required to repeat back a string of digits or numbers after they've been read to you at a rate of about one a second. That capacity can't be improved no matter how much you practice. It is part of the brain's memory

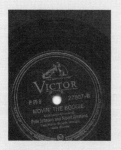

Frontal-Lobe Flexibility Builder
A perspective-switching game to help your
creative thinking skills:

**How many grooves are on one side of
a 33 rpm phonograph record?**

Creative Thinking Quiz
These brain teasers help to give your creative thinking skills a
jump-start by challenging you to think about solutions on multiple levels. Are the following statements true or false?

This statement is false.

Their are four errers in this sentence.

(See page 44 for the solutions)

"chip," the raw brain power; a kind of IQ-like intelli-
gence-in-isolation.

Of course, the kind of short-term capacity measured by
the digit span test isn't what we normally think of as
memory or long-term learning. How well you remember the plot of a movie, or somebody's name, or the
sequence of all the U.S. presidents does not depend on
short-term capacity. What counts more is whether you
have the mental stamina or discipline to study such
things, whether you're interested in them, whether
you're motivated to pay attention, how wide-spread
your general historical knowledge is, and on and on.

**Yes, with age the brain's processing speed slows
down, along with short-term capacity, but . . .**
. . . what doesn't have to get worse with age are skills
that contribute to a good memory.

Study habits: When students develop good study habits that help them learn more things in less time, they don't improve mental processing speed. They do learn techniques that help them to take maximal advantage of whatever information processing capacity they have. Those capacities that influence the ability to learn — interest, discipline, motivation, general knowledge — all *can* be improved. Those attitudes and habits can translate into a stronger memory. Those are the true memory muscles that you can strengthen.

Making an effort: Your brain is your best friend, but it can be lazy. It is about the size of a three-pound grapefruit but it burns about 20 percent of the body's supply of nutrient glucose in the blood. So it shuts itself down when it is not made to work — just as you save heating costs by turning off the radiators and closing down rooms in a big house if you are not living in them. Anybody who tackles a challenging mental task, and keeps at it, feels tired at the end even though they haven't put out any physical effort greater than, say, typing into a computer.

Brain cells have "fingers" that project off the dendrites. Those fingers reach out to connect to other cells in order to complete a circuit to get things done, like learning something, for example. When the brain shuts down those connections withdraw. Weak connections, weak memory.

The good news: When you make an effort to figure out something and learn about it your brain fires up — especially the hippocampus and parts that perform analytical executive functions in your frontal lobes. Those neurons grow new "fingers" on the dendrites right

(See page 42)

Frontal-Lobe Flexibility Builder Solution

Only one (one continuous spiral groove).

Creative Thinking Quiz Solution

You cannot really call either statement true or false without encountering a contradiction. For the first one, if you say the statement is true, then the problem is that the statement itself claims to be *false.* If, on the other hand, you say the statement is false, the problem is that the statement itself makes that same claim. For the second one, the three (not four) spelling errors might lead you to believe that the statement is false. In that case, though, the very claim to contain four (not three) errors is also an error, which might make you think the statement is true. But in *that* case, the claim to contain four errors is false. The point with these brain teasers is not to get the right answer, but to run through the logical entailments so that you see the paradoxes. Both run you around in circles, but get your brain going.

away so they can get the job done. With that new connection capacity, processes like memory storage and retrieval become easier and work faster.

In fact, as the information becomes more firmly entrenched in your store of knowledge your frontal lobes no longer have to work as hard when you're using or accessing it. Brain regions further back, where the knowledge is actually stored, become activated. This frees "executive" capacities in the frontal lobes to do what they do best: evaluate the usefulness of incoming data, plan ahead, set goals, imagine the steps necessary to reach those goals, control inappropriate emotional responses, apply logical reasoning to solve problems — and all the other skills that separate humans from other animals.

Healthy frontal lobes never lose their ability to learn even though they may slow down

As researchers have shown in brain scan studies testing older adults vs. college students, the cells in frontal lobes do tend to change with age in ways that require more effort to goad them into action. This part of the brain is the most recently evolved part of the human brain.

It is the last to grow fully mature (at about 18 years old) and it is the first part to begin to slow its processing with age.

On the other hand, the older you get the more time and opportunity you've had to accumulate knowledge. That's important because the more information you have in memory, the easier it is to learn more new things. The frontal lobes are crucial to relating something new to something familiar. That is one of the main tricks to remembering something new. The ability to make those associations consciously is part of its job. It notes what episodes and things fit into which categories, i.e. faces, tools, foods, tastes, smells, sounds, etc. Its ability to "tag" new short-term memories by the categories it fits into makes up most of its day as the brain's "executive."

Luckily, some learning and memory systems don't demand conscious effort

For example, you spend a week in Rio without really trying to speak Portuguese. Even so you learn the

45

Portuguese words for "hello" without much effort. This happens automatically because you want to learn it. It is a goal. So you pay attention when you hear others speaking. You hear it frequently and you get to practice it, sometimes with pronunciation help from a native. Acquiring most new information, however, is harder work because you have to create your own motivation, strategies, and learning atmosphere.

Also, your primitive emotional memory systems often sear experiences into your brain instantly and permanently, whether asked to or not. Subtle rewards and punishments nudge human behavior this way or that unconsciously, just as Pavlov's dog learned to salivate when he heard the dinner bell. Humans even share with sea slugs and fruit flies some of the instinctive learning systems located way down in the most primitive part of their brain stems. But, for most of the things humans want consciously to remember, their recently evolved frontal lobes, located just above their eyes, must kick into gear.

A real life example of the-more-you-know-the-easier-it-is-to-learn-and-remember-new-stuff

If you already know French, it's easier to learn Portuguese. And even if you don't know French, Portuguese is easier for you to learn than Korean, because there are more similarities between English and Portuguese than between English and Korean. When you want to learn something new you always have to put more effort into switching on your frontal lobes, but they don't have to work as hard when you can relate the new knowledge to something else you already know.

The Most Important Take-home Lesson

If you make the initial effort to embed new facts into knowledge networks you already have, you are reducing the amount of effort you have to make in the long run to be able to remember and use those facts. In effect, you are setting things up so that in the future your brain can do the work for you. But you have to make the initial effort! That is crucial. When you do, this is how your brain lights up.

1. FIRST EXPERIENCE. Most fade quickly. To transfer to long-term memory, you need to pay attention and make a point of remembering.

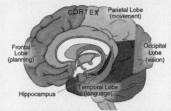

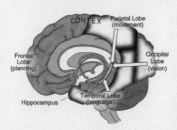

2. CONSOLIDATION. Strengthening of pathways connecting points of brain activity, creating a network of activity corresponding to the original experience. Hippocampus plays an important role in creating and strengthening the connections. Sleep is a crucial part of this step. Consolidation is not all or nothing. You don't wake up the morning after learning something with a permanent new memory. You have to come back to it repeatedly and use it.

3. RECALL. In the future, you can reactivate the network on command. Frontal cortex tells the hippocampus to activate the network.

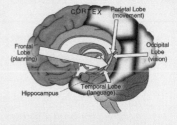

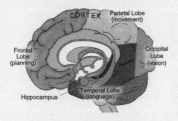

4. KNOWLEDGE. As the memory becomes very well integrated into your semantic store, the hippocampus and frontal cortex are less and less necessary to reactivate the network.

A Tip-of the-Tongue Test

Do I need to remember what the capital of France is? No, I don't. It doesn't matter to me if I remember what the capital of France is, because I *already know* the capital is Paris. Do you remember your name? How to open a door? How to drive? Many, many routine parts of your knowledge base have moved into your brain's storehouse of knowledge. You can access them so effortlessly you hardly have to use your frontal lobes at all. Long ago in your life your frontal lobes recruited memory systems to switch facts and procedures like those from "memories" to "knowledge" by connecting new information to what you already know. You linked something new to something familiar — something you know you won't forget.

But sometimes, you can't bring up some bit of old knowledge — why?

Usually it is a name for something. Exasperating, isn't it? The technical term is "blocking." Your mind lost the linkage temporarily. Stress or environmental distractions can cause that. A better name for this problem is "tip-of-the-tongue." Often another word that is almost the correct one comes up and gets in the way. All you know is that it isn't exactly the correct

More steps to a better memory:

Develop an "attitude"

The first two steps to remember things better are to pay attention and take an active role in making sense of things by relating them to things you already know. There is another step. Really, what you're doing when you put out that kind of effort is changing your attitude toward what's around you and toward your own mind. This kind of attitude shift helps when you want to answer. (When that happens the best strategy often is to change the subject, let your subconscious dampen the interloper and start searching for the correct name. For that reason, crossword puzzle mavens often move to another part of the grid, or even walk away for a while when they are "blocking" on a word.)

The Test:

Here are some links that should prompt an answer or, maybe, a block. We supplied the correct answer for the first one so you can see how it works. See page 55 for the answers.

France + capital = ? ("Paris" of course.)

Movie actor + "Frankly, I don't give a damn" =?

Pencil + pointing-machine = ?

Verdi + opera = ?

London + river = ?

Potatoes + crispy-thin = ?

President + Desert Storm = ?

Perhaps you never knew some of these answers but you may block on others. To help with those, here are some additional links for those blocked questions, but these are scrambled up: Scarlet, Iraq, salty, electric, Egypt, Big Ben.

You see how the mind finds facts?

remember something important (where you left your pocketbook or what your boss told you to tell the new client) as well as when you want to remember something that is, by itself, trivial and uninteresting (the number on your hotel room door).

Use proven tricks

People who use *mnemonic* (memorization) tricks often *seem* to have a better memory even though the trick does not change the way their brain stores data. The "salesman's" trick, for example, is to immediately repeat the name of a person he has just met several times in conversation. Hearing it in his mind's ear helps to consolidate the name in his memory. (For another name-memorizing trick, see Self-test, page 33.)

Other memory aids

Similarly, "crutches" help a memorization ability that is less than perfect — always putting keys in the same place, or making a written list of the things to do that day. Such mnemonic tricks that improve everyday performance do not, as a rule, improve the brain's capacity to store and recall data but, with use, the tricks become automatic and habitual. That path to a "better" memory can affect daily life for the better in many practical ways. The psychological boost of seeing memory improve can also boost self-confidence which, in turn, empowers the will to tackle a new and different challenge in life.

Cultivate self-efficacy and coherence

Self-efficacy is very important for brain health. It is essentially a sense of being in control of one's own life circumstances. Older people who rate high in self-efficacy also rate high in memory, on average. This kind of attitude affects other aspects of health, too. Older adults with a strong sense of *coherence* — a sense of confidence that their life circumstances are manageable, controllable, and meaningful — have stronger immune systems and better health overall. A recent study found that among older adults who were being relocated to new housing — a situation that's stressful for almost anyone — the ones with the highest sense of coherence scores also had the lowest drop in immune system cell count.

Self-efficacy and sense of coherence extend to your attitude toward your own brain, too. It's crucially important to believe that you have some understanding of how your brain works, what might harm it, and what can keep it healthy. That will give you a sense of control over what is, after all, your most vital possession. A feeling of confidence in your ability to maintain your cognitive faculties can become a self-justifying belief.

Avoid situations that make you feel stressed and helpless day after day

On many levels and in many ways, attitude can empower or corrode your brain. Constant stress can be harmful (see Common Substances That May Harm the Brain, page 78). Stress hormones called *cortisol* will kill neurons in the hippocampus that allow it to direct short-term knowledge into memory. But it's really not a hectic life or occasions that you "get up for" to perform well that constitute "stress" in the relevant sense. Stress is harmful when it takes the form of a feeling of being overwhelmed and out of control. It's actually that subjective attitude that leads to a cascade of physical responses that can harm your brain.

Try to cultivate mental flexibility

Along with the executive skills described above, older people tend to have a harder time with mental flexibility. This skill is needed to switch problem-solving strategies in midstream as the problem itself evolves or the incoming data you had planned for start to change. For example, a traffic holdup on a route from home to a favorite restaurant may make it sensible to change to another route. A business strategy may have to be switched around to reflect feedback from the market.

Divergent vs. Literal Thinking

Tasks that require divergent thinking (see Section 4, page 132), on the other hand, test imagination, originality, fluency, and flexibility of thought, rather than the ability to come up with one right answer. If asked to name as many uses as you can think of for a hammer, the potential list is endless. A good response could be scored in terms of quantity — how many uses can be described in a minute — or quality — how unusual or imaginative the uses are. ("Drive a nail into wood" is obvious; "crack walnuts" is a little less so; and "lean it against an unlockable door to sound an alarm if someone walks into the room at night" would be the least obvious of all.) Divergent ability depends on frontal lobe regions that also support planning and reasoning about possible future events. If these regions are damaged, creative divergent-thinking ability may be impaired even if IQ remains perfectly intact.

Traditional tests of intelligence and cognitive fitness do not test for this kind of adaptability, inventiveness, creativity, and mental flexibility.

Many older people, as well as patients with frontal-lobe brain damage persevere with a habitual sequence of behaviors even though they have become obviously useless or even harmful. Appropriately, this condition is called *perseveration*. Perseveration problems that come with normal aging reveal a loss of mental flexibility that may benefit from some of the training methods presented in the next two chapters.

Mental flexibility can be cultivated with practice
Like many creative intellectual abilities that correlate with success in real-world tasks, mental flexibility and the knack for spotting similarities between two different objects, situations, or events are not measured by traditional IQ tests. This kind of *divergent intelligence* is distinct from the *convergent* thinking measured by most intelligence tests. A prime example of convergent thinking is deductive logic, as in this famous syllogism: *All men are mortal; Socrates is a man; therefore, Socrates is mortal*. With convergent-thinking problems, there is always supposed to be a unique solution (*"Socrates is mortal"*) that the available information leads you to.

Can we protect against the effects of aging on memory?

> ❝When I was young I could remember everything, whether it happened or not. Now that I am older I can remember only those things that never happened. ❞
>
> *Mark Twain*

The kinds of memory loss that begin afflicting people as they approach old age can be traced to physical changes in their brains. The frontal-lobe skills (such as executive and task management skills, elaborative encoding, and divergent thinking), are some of the hardest to acquire early in life, are acquired more slowly than many other cognitive skills, and are the easiest to lose later in life.

The brain is like the rest of the body. With age the muscles of the limbs lose mass. However, exercises can build back lost mass. In fact, the results are most dramatic when the muscles have become most flabby. It will never equal the mass of youth, but the change in size and strength is clearly noticeable in a short time. Similarly, mental skills that are slow to develop and have rusted from neglect can often be readily improved as well. The cognitive skills that are easiest to lose are also the most improvable with practice. For example, the best way to be an expert at organizing information and using it to your advantage is to work at it, consistently and often.

Brain-training techniques

Determination: The crucial first step to brain-training is to respect your own ability to take on new challenges. What is the worst that could happen if you picked up a musical instrument you used to play, or joined a book discussion group, or sat down to learn the basics of statistics, or started a modest business with a friend or relative, or joined a committee in municipal government, or stopped to plan professional goals at some point in the future to avoid being painted into a corner?

Getting better at solving puzzles: The best kind of paper-and-pencil puzzles target a variety of mental

faculties related to practical, real-world situations.
It is more important to develop skills in the areas you
find hardest at first. Those are the ones that stimulate
brain circuits you do not normally use. But you need
them too, because most real-world situations require
a wide variety of brain circuits to handle them effectively. Mental and other physical conditioning
demand more practice and effort at first when you
are 70 than it did at 30. But, somehow, the rewards
are sweeter, especially when they build confidence in
managing the challenges of life rather than being
managed *by* them.

Is there any way that memorization and problem-
solving techniques can actually protect or promote
the brain's health and agility? For simple tricks like
always putting keys in the same place, the answer is
probably no. For more cognitively complex skills, the
answer is yes. The very process of figuring out new
and effective problem-solving techniques when needed is, itself, rigorous exercise of mental skills and
helps keep the brain functional and fit. The next two
chapters show how engaging tasks, games, and puzzles can be a crucial part of an "enriched environment" program that may actually help the brain grow
new brain connections and protect the ones it
already has.

Answers to Tip-of the-Tongue Test, page 49:
Sharpener, Thames, George Bush, Clark Gable, *Aida*, Chips

References for Section 1

Brain changes with normal aging:

Albert, M.S., and M.B. Moss. 1996. "Neuropsychology of aging: findings in humans and monkeys." In E. Schneider and J.W. Rowe (eds.), *The Handbook of the Biology of Aging,* 4th ed. San Diego: Academic Press.

Bryan, J., and M.A. Luszcz. 1996. "Speed of information processing as a mediator between age and free-recall performance." *Psychology and Aging* 18/3:383-93.

Craik, F.I.M., et al. 1995. "Memory changes in normal aging." In A.D. Baddeley, B.A. Wilson, and F. N. Watt (eds.), *Handbook of Memory Disorders*. New York: Wiley.

Crawford, S., and S Channon. 2002. "Dissociation between performance on abstract tests of executive function and problem solving in real-life-type situations in normal aging." *Aging and Mental Health* 6/1:12-21.

Daigneault, S., and C.M.J. Braun. 1993. "Working memory and the self-ordered pointing task: further evidence of early prefrontal decline in normal aging." *Journal of Clinical and Experimental Neuropsychology* 15:881-95.

Fillit, H.M., et al. 2002. "Achieving and maintaining cognitive vitality with aging." *Mayo Clinic Proceedings* 77/7:681-96.

Grady, C.L., et al. 1995. "Age-related reductions in human recognition memory due to impaired encoding." *Science* 269:218-21.

Guttmann, C.R., et al. 1998. "White matter changes with normal aging." *Neurology* 50/4:972-8.

Hartman, M., and L. Hasher. 1991. "Aging and suppression: memory for previously relevant information." *Psychology and Aging* 6:587-94.

Hasher, L., et al. 1991. "Age and inhibition." *Journal of Experimental Psychology: Learning, Memory, and Cognition* 17:163-9.

Logan, J.M., et al. 2002. "Under-recruitment and nonselective recruitment: dissociable neural mechanisms associated with aging." *Neuron* 33/5:827-40.

Luszcz, M.A., and J. Bryan. 1999. "Toward understanding age-related memory loss in late adulthood." *Gerontology* 45:2-9.

Moscovitch, M., and G. Winocur. 1992. "The neuropsychology of memory and aging." In F.I.M. Craik and T.A. Salthouse (eds.), *The Handbook of Aging and Cognition*. Hillsdale, N.J.: Erlbaum, 315–72.

Myerson, J., et al. 1992. "General slowing in semantic priming and word recognition." *Psychology and Aging* 7:257-70.

Park, D.C., et al. 1996. "Mediators of long-term memory performance across the life span." *Psychology and Aging* 11:621-37.

Parkin, A.J., and B.M. Walter. 1992. "Recollective experience, normal aging, and frontal dysfunction." *Psychology and Aging* 2:290-8.

Peters, A. 2002. "Structural changes that occur during normal aging of primate cerebral hemispheres." *Neuroscience and Biobehavioral Reviews* 26/7:733-41.

Salthouse, T.A. 1996. "General and specific speed mediation of adult age differences in memory." *Journals of Gerontology, Series B: Psychological Sciences and Social Sciences* 51B:P30-42.

Salthouse, T.A. 1996. "The processing-speed theory of adult age differences in cognition." *Psychological Review* 10:403-28.

Schacter, D.L. 1996. *Searching for Memory.* New York: Basic Books.

Schretlen, D., et al. 2000. "Evaluating the contributions of processing speed, executive ability, and frontal lobe volume to normal age-related differences in fluid intelligence." *Journal of the International Neuropsychological Society* 6/1:52-61.

Simensky, J.D., and N. Abeles. 2002. "Decline in verbal memory performance with advancing age: the role of frontal lobe functioning." *Aging and Mental Health* 6/3: 293-303.

Small, S.A., et al. 2002. "Imaging hippocampal function across the human life span: is memory decline normal or not?" *Annals of Neurology* 51/3:290-5.

Volkow, N.D., et al. 2000. "Association between age-related decline in brain dopamine activity and impairment in frontal and cingulate metabolism." *American Journal of Psychiatry* 157/1: 75-80.

West, R.L. 1996. "An application of prefrontal cortex function theory to cognitive aging." *Psychological Bulletin* 120:272-92.

Woodruff-Pak, D.D. 1997. *The Neuropsychology of Aging.* Oxford: Blackwell.

Differences between normal aging and Alzheimer's:

Albert, M.S., et al. 2001. "Preclinical prediction of AD using neuropsychological tests." *Journal of the International Neuropsychological Society* 7/5:631-9.

Chodosh, J., et al. 2002. "Predicting cognitive impairment in high-functioning community-dwelling older persons: MacArthur Studies of Successful Aging." *Journal of the American Geriatric Society* 50/6:1051-60.

Garraux, G., et al. 1999. "Comparison of impaired subcortico-frontal metabolic networks in normal aging, subcortico-frontal dementia, and cortical frontal dementia." *Neuroimage* 10/2:149-62.

Kensinger, E.A., et al. 2002. "Effects of normal aging and Alzheimer's disease on emotional memory." *Emotion* 2/2:118-34.

Morrison, J.H., and P.R. Hof. 2002. "Selective vulnerability of corticocortical and hippocampal circuits in aging and Alzheimer's disease." *Progress in Brain Research* 136:467-86.

Sliwinski, M., and H. Buschke. 1997. "Processing speed and memory in aging and dementia." *Journal of Gerontology: Psychological Sciences* 52B/6:P308-18.

Sperling, R.A., et al. 2003. "fMRI studies of associative encoding in young and elderly controls and mild Alzheimer's disease." *Journal of Neurology, Neurosurgery, and Psychiatry* 74/1:44-50.

Role of enriched environment in brain maintenance:
Friedland, R.P., et al. 2001. "Patients with Alzheimer's disease have reduced activities in midlife compared with healthy control-group members." *Proceedings of the National Academy of Sciences* USA98/6:3440-5.

Shimamura, A.P., et al. 1995. "Memory and cognitive abilities in university professors: evidence for successful aging." *Psychological Science* 6/5:271-7.

Wilson, R.S., et al. 2002. "Cognitive activity and incident AD in a population-based sample of older persons." *Neurology* 59/12:1910-14.

Wilson, R.S., et al. 2002. "Participation in cognitively stimulating activities and risk of incident Alzheimer's disease." *JAMA* 287/6:742-8.

Neurogenesis:
Kuhn, H.G., T.D. Palmer, and E. Fuchs. 2001. "Adult neurogenesis: a compensatory mechanism for neuronal damage." *European Archives of* 251/4:152-8.

General learning and memory:

Baddeley, A. 1986. "Working Memory." Oxford: Clarendon Press.

Bartsch, D., et al. 1995. "Aplysia CREB2 represses long-term facilitation." *Cell* 83:979-92.

Bechara, A., et al. 1996. "Failure to respond autonomically to anticipated future outcomes following damage to prefrontal cortex." *Cerebral Cortex* 6:215-25.

Buckner, R.L., and M.E. Wheeler. 2001. "The cognitive neuroscience of remembering." *Nature Reviews* 2/9:624-34.

Grabowski T.J., H. Damasio, and A.R. Damasio. 1998. "Premotor and prefrontal correlates of category-related lexical retrieval." *Neuroimage* 7/3:232-43.

Loftus, E.F., and J.E. Pickrell. 1995. "The formation of false memories." *Psychiatric Annals* 25:720-5.

Lezak, M.D. 1995. *Neuropsychological Assessment,* 3rd ed. New York: Oxford University Press.

Rapp, S., G. Brenes, and A.P. Marsh. 2002. "Memory enhancement training for older adults with mild cognitive impairment: a preliminary study." *Aging and Mental Health* 6/1: 5-11.

Shallice, T., and P. Burgess. 1996. "The domain of supervisory processes and temporal organization of behaviour." *Philosophical Transactions of the Royal Society of London* B 351:1405-12.

Shimamura, A.B. 1995. "Memory and frontal lobe function." In M.S. Gazzaniga (ed.), *The Cognitive Neurosciences.* Cambridge MA: MIT Press, 803-13.

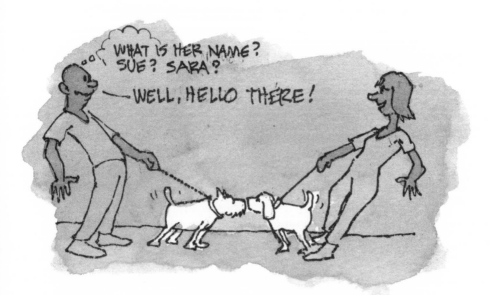

COMMON COGNITIVE PROBLEMS AND WHAT YOU CAN DO ABOUT THEM

HOW ARE YOU DOING?

EVALUATING THE SOURCES OF COGNITIVE PROBLEMS

COMMON SUBSTANCES THAT MAY HARM THE BRAIN

How Are You Doing?

We are all aware of the problems faced by a graying society as the baby boomer demographic bulge moves towards retirement age. With the increasing numbers of old people, health care costs are starting to spiral. One of the most urgent health care concerns these days is Alzheimer's disease (AD). Just thirty years ago that form of dementia was considered a rarity. Now, four million people have it in the U.S. alone. According to public health authorities, that translates into an annual financial burden of $100 billion. We can predict that, over the next twenty years, the numbers of people with the disease, and with it the financial burden, will go up by a factor of three.

On a more personal level, each one of us finds it unbearable that, simply by aging, we could lose our enjoyment of life, our memory, our identity. Fortunately, research into the biochemistry of aging and technology for manipulating that process is advancing rapidly. New technologies allow researchers to watch what parts of a living human brain are activated when its owner responds to test questions. Research results are accumulating daily. We're learning about new roles for the brain's chemical messengers, about how groups of brain cells work together to process information, about the actions of stress hormones, growth hormones, and other crucially important elements of the brain's complex and flexible support system.

It has become possible for scientists to identify specific genes that trigger memory storage, addiction, and other responses to the environment. These discoveries are being published in scientific journals today; they will change the way humans live in the next generation. But what can we do now? The baby boomer generation is turning 50 years old at the rate of six people per second as you read this. What can they do now to keep their lives interesting as their old age stretches out before them? How can they avoid losing their awareness of themselves and becoming an institutionalized burden on their families?

What are the signs of Alzheimer's disease?
Even though AD can be a devastating disease, its early symptoms are subtle and easy to overlook. In fact, in its early stages the signs of AD look a lot like the changes that come with ordinary aging —sometimes known as "benign senescent forgetfulness." It's often only when AD is more advanced that it becomes obvious that something is wrong.

That poses a challenge for AD treatment, because whatever modest success has been achieved thus far in slowing the progress of AD works best in the early stages of the disease. As new, more effective treatments are developed it will become even more important to have a way of diagnosing AD before it has made destructive inroads on an afflicted brain. As with most diseases, treatments that may be effective in avoiding or forestalling AD in its early stages may not work well once the disease has become more advanced.

Even better than having highly accurate means of diagnosing incipient AD would be techniques for identifying AD before it shows any outward signs at all. Researchers are using neuroimaging technology such as MRI, PET, and SPECT to search for possible signs of Alzheimer's in the brain — what they call "preclinical predictors" — before there's been any measurable falloff in memory or reasoning. As yet, though, there is no single test that can confirm an AD diagnosis. Instead, a diagnosis of AD can be made with up to 90 percent accuracy by systematically using a battery of tests to rule out other possible causes of progressive cognitive decline one by one.

Just as early signs of AD are easy to dismiss as harmless signs of aging, symptoms that provoke anxiety about dementia may in fact be perfectly normal. All old people tend to experience memory loss or forgetfulness, occasional difficulty remembering a word or a name and difficulty learning new tasks (how to use a personal computer, for example). How do you know if middle-aged and older people who are perfectly healthy are misinterpreting insignificant mental lapses as dementia symptoms? The following chart, compiled by the Alzheimer's Association, describes some of the most useful points of distinction between normal aging and dementia. Keep in mind that the chart is less useful for identifying very early AD than it is for identifying the disease in its more advanced stages.

What are the risk factors?

The single most important risk factor for AD is age. At age 65, only about two out of one hundred people have serious mental disabilities that turn out to be AD. By age 80, some current research shows that the ratio rises to at least twenty in one hundred — one in five. By age 90, about half of all people have the disease. Four million older, adult Americans now have AD, and as the over-65 population increases over the next twenty years, the number is expected to triple.

Genes

Neuroscientific research has revealed that there may be a genetic component to AD, although genetic predisposition is a much weaker risk factor than age. Many studies of identical twins prove that genes aren't the whole story because even when both twins do get it, often many years intervene between onset in twin #1 and twin #2. The fact that a parent or brother or sister has had AD does not mean that another sibling will also end up getting it. Many people who have genes that raise their Alzheimer's risk never get AD at all even if they live to an advanced age. People who lack a genetically "risky" profile, conversely, may still develop AD in spite of their genes. So you might view the genetic risk for Alzheimer's as somewhat like the increased risk for skin cancer among people with blond hair, blue eyes, and a fair complexion.

Genes play a more significant role in a small percentage of people who have the early-onset form of AD, about 40 percent of whom have a family history of the disease. The early-onset form of AD, however, is relatively rare.

Normal Aging versus Dementia

Very early symptoms of progressive dementia, including AD, are mild — the sort of forgetfulness common among most older people, and even among some middle-aged ones. As the disease progresses, it becomes more easily distinguished from simple benign forgetfulness.

	Normal	Dementia
1) **Memory loss at work**	Occasionally forgetting an assignment, deadline, or colleague's name	Frequent forgetfulness and unexplainable confusion
2) **Difficulty with familiar tasks**	Occasional distractedness — forgetting to serve a dish that was intended to be included with a meal, for example	Severe forgetfulness — forgetting that you made a meal at all, for example
3) **Language impairment**	Occasional difficulty finding the right word	Frequent and severe difficulty finding the right word, resulting in speech that does not make sense
4) **Disorientation**	Occasionally forgetting the day of the week	Becoming lost on the way to the store
5) **Judgment problems**	Choosing an outfit that turns out to be somewhat warm or cold for the weather — neglecting to bring a sweater to a baseball game on a cool September evening, for example	Dressing blatantly inappropriately — for example, wearing several layers of warm clothing on a hot summer day

	Normal	Alzheimer's
6) Abstract thinking difficulties	Occasional difficulty balancing a checkbook accurately	Inability to perform basic calculations, such as subtracting a check for $40 from a balance of $280
7) Misplacing objects	Misplacing keys or a wallet from time to time	Putting things in inappropriate places — a wallet in the oven, for example
8) Mood or behavior changes	Changes in mood from day to day	Rapid, dramatic mood swings with no apparent cause
9) Personality changes	Moderate personality change with age	Dramatic and disturbing personality change — for example, a traditionally easygoing person becoming hostile or angry
10) Reduced initiative	Temporarily tiring of social obligations or household chores	Permanent loss of interest in many or all social activities or chores

(Source: Alzheimer's Association Web site: www.alz.org.)

Indeed, one of the reasons that most people hadn't heard much about Alzheimer's disease until about thirty years ago is that the early twentieth-century pioneering research of Alois Alzheimer (after whom the disease is named) focused on the early-onset form. Until recently, most people died before they could get the much more common late-onset type of AD. Even then, if symptoms of the late-onset form did develop, they were often viewed as normal and inevitable signs of aging, rather than as an expression of a disease.

EVALUATING THE SOURCES OF COGNITIVE PROBLEMS

If there is even suspicion of a problem

Should there be concern about possible dementia in a friend or relative, make an appointment with a physician or psychologist trained in neuro-diagnosis. The physician will want details about the kinds of behavior that raised concern, so make notes of specific changes in behavior and take them along. On the first visit some physicians prefer not to examine the subject but to interview only those people who have observed the patient closely, especially if they have done so over a long period of time. Close friends and family members will often be more aware of, and more concerned about, memory lapses and signs of cognitive confusion than a person suffering from dementia.

The next step a physician or other professional advisor will take is to administer a mental status examination to the patient in order to get objective confirmation of cognitive difficulties, followed by physical and neuro-logical examinations. Standard mental status examinations evaluate short-term memory, ability to pay attention to and follow simple directions, the ability to copy simple line drawings, and the like. In fact, the tasks in such standardized tests of mental status are so easy that difficulty answering even a small percentage of the questions indicates a likely cognitive problem.

If the results of the clinical examination test of mental status indicate a problem, the next step is to investigate the possibility of traumatic brain damage such as ministrokes or a brain tumor. It is standard practice to take a complete medical history and to review the medical record for other possible causes of mental confusion that may be treated directly. Among the many causes of symptoms similar to those typical of dementia are side effects of prescription medications and over-the-counter medicine, vitamin deficiency, thyroid problems, alcohol abuse, and diet. The symptoms of depression can mimic those of dementia. Depression is common among elderly people who may feel vulnerable, useless, lonely, or embarrassed by physical or mental disabilities. Unlike dementia, however, depression is readily 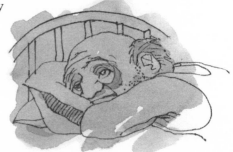 treated with lifestyle changes or medication.

Eventually, if there is clear-cut cognitive decline and all the other possible causes have been ruled out, a tentative diagnosis of AD may be reached.

If the signs of cognitive decline are professionally diagnosed as AD, even though no cure is yet known, there are treatments that may slow the progression of the disease. In addition, ongoing clinical trials of the effectiveness of currently available drugs and nutritional supplements, as well as trials of new drugs that aren't yet FDA-approved, are definitely worth following, preferably with the help of a health care professional knowledgeable about them.

Is it dementia? Or could it be depression?

The relationship between depression and dementia, including AD, is complex. Depression is common in AD patients. A recent brain-scan study showed decreased activity in the frontal lobes of depressed AD patients. There are two ways of looking at these results. One explanation is that depression could well be a symptom of the cluster of brain changes brought about by the disease. It may also in some cases be an emotional response to a conscious fear of cognitive decline. Many researchers suspect that depression may be a risk factor for the gradual onset of dementia. Some studies even appear to show that people with a history of depression are at greater risk for AD.

On the other hand, the symptoms of depression have a lot in common with the early symptoms of AD. Some of the most common symptoms of depression also occur in AD. Inattentiveness, disorientation, forgetfulness, and mental lethargy are frequently reported in both conditions. To compound the confusion between the symptoms, all of them can be especially pronounced in depressed older people. In fact, they resemble the cognitive impairments of AD so closely that the two can be very difficult to tell apart, even for a trained medical professional (see pages 74 to 76).

Unlike true AD symptoms, the dementia-like symptoms of depression are relatively treatable and reversible. Depression often follows withdrawal from social, mental, and physical stimulation, especially in older people. This kind of withdrawal, which is very likely to occur when one retires from work, can be described as retirement syndrome. Unfortunately, when they retire, many people lose their motivation to tax their brains. They lose many of their social contacts as well as their urgent need to analyze and solve thorny problems of the sort that may have arisen regularly in the normal course of a working day. Unless replaced with the cognitive challenges of other active interests and social interactions, the cost of a relaxed retirement may be the beginning of noticeable cognitive impairment. Depression may therefore result from an isolated, routine lifestyle having an effect on the chemical messenger systems within the brain. There have been rapid advances in the development of drugs that can help to balance the messenger systems involved in depression, so it's important to diagnose and treat it.

Symptoms caused by the side effects of medication
As bodies age, they function less well. Old injuries or other conditions start acting up. Older people start taking more medications to relieve new aches and inconveniences. Most medications cause side effects, some of which produce the same medical and emotional symptoms caused by physical deterioration of brain circuits. Older bodies become less efficient at getting rid of the medications after they have had their beneficial effects. Older people tend to take more medications than younger people, especially sleeping pills and drugs for

heart disease, which often cause dementia-like symptoms, especially if several of them are taken together. If
mental decline is due to medication alternatives might
be considered.

Sleeping pills, for example, are common culprits in
medication-induced mental confusion. Sleeping pill
abuse is often a result of depression, because poor sleep
and depression often go hand in hand in the elderly.
Lifestyle causes of depression, such as social, mental,
and physical inactivity, can cause sleep problems as
well. Antidepressant medications can cause forgetfulness, disorientation, and inattentiveness in some people. A program of increasing social, mental and
physical stimulation, known as *environmental
enrichment*, may often be effective in combating both
depression and the dementia-like symptoms caused by
medication use.

In extreme cases, alcoholism may lead to Wernicke-
Korsakoff syndrome, an irreversible disorder with symptoms of amnesia and confusion. More commonly,
excessive alcohol consumption for a decade or more
can cause an AD-like dementia marked by memory, orientation, and attention impairments. This kind of alco-
hol-induced dementia is at least partly reversible.

Small strokes can cause dementia
Tiny strokes, sometimes called "mini-strokes," are
caused by small interruptions in the supply of blood to
groups of brain cells, producing a small area of dead
brain tissue, known as an *infarct*. A sufficient accumulation of tiny strokes can cause what's called *multi-infarct*

Delayed Recall

Several versions of delayed word recall test have been used to help distinguish people with early Alzheimer's from those who are just depressed.

In this version, there are two shopping lists (Monday and Tuesday). What you are going to try to do is memorize the items on each list, first Monday and then Tuesday.

It helps to have an "examiner" for this. If you do not, just follow the instructions for the examiner and cover up the list as you write down your answers.

Monday	*Tuesday*
oranges	bananas
wrench	corkscrew
rosemary	peppercorns
pineapple	apples
thumbtacks	can opener
socks	oysters
salt	basil
swimsuit	sardines
hammer	mixing bowl
grapes	lemons
paprika	bay leaf
sandals	tuna
plums	apricots
oregano	cinnamon
t-shirt	measuring cup
shovel	flounder

Examiner:

1) Read these instructions out loud to the person taking the test:

   "I am going to read you a shopping list. Pay attention, because as soon as I'm done reading the list I want you to repeat back to me as many of the items as you can remember, in any order you like."

2) Then, read the Monday list out loud, slowly and clearly, about one word per second.

3) As soon as you are done reading the list, ask the test-taker to recite out loud as many items from the list as possible, writing down each item as the test-taker names it. Once the test-taker cannot recall any more items, read Monday's list out loud once more, and ask him or her once again to recite as many as possible, including ones already recited the first time. Repeat this procedure three more times, for a total of five run-throughs.

4) Next, read the following instructions:
   "I'm now going to read you a different list. Pay attention clearly so you remember as many of the items as possible."

5) Then, read Tuesday's list out loud, slowly and clearly. Once you are done, ask the test-taker to recall as many items from the list as possible, but this time do it only once. Then, ask the test-taker once again to recall as many items from Monday's list as possible, writing down the answers as they are recited.

6) Finally, after a delay of thirty minutes, ask the test-taker once again to recite as many items as possible from the first (Monday's) list.

(continued on page 76)

Scoring norms for people under 65 years old:
After the first run-through of the list:
    5 items or under remembered from the first list: Needs work
    6-8 words: Good
    9-10 words: Excellent
    11+ : Extraordinary

After the fifth run-through:
    10 or under: Needs work
    11-12: Good
    13-14: Excellent
    15-16: Extraordinary

These norms fall off with age. Women also perform better than men, on average. This might be because women seem to be better at organizing the list using categories, for example by putting all the fruit together. This makes it easier for them to remember the list. Psychologists call this a "semantic clustering" strategy. However, the use of a semantic clustering strategy also tends to fall off with age. Older people tend to make more errors of falsely supplying a word that was not on the list. These intrusion errors include interference errors, such as reciting some of the first list's items in recall of the second list (proactive interference), or the second list's items in the recall of the first list (retroactive interference). You may want to refer back to the discussion of these terms in more detail in Chapter 2.

Scoring norms for people with Alzheimer's:
People with early-stage Alzheimer's tend to recall hardly any items on the first trial, and only about five to six items on the fifth trial. Alzheimer's patients also tend to make far more intrusion errors (over one third of their responses tend to be words that did not appear on the actual list) than healthy people of the same age. Also, they tend to forget most of the items on the list in the delayed recall stage (after 30 minutes), unlike healthy people of the same age, who recall most of them.

dementia. Some mini-strokes, also known as transient ischemic attacks (TIAs), are so small that they often go unnoticed. In fact, they can't even be seen in a brain scan. However, a sufficient accumulation even of TIAs can lead to symptoms of dementia. While multi-infarct dementia isn't as easily treated as dementia caused by depression, medication, or alcohol, reducing high blood pressure can often help avoid future mini-strokes.

COMMON SUBSTANCES THAT MAY HARM THE BRAIN

How to help your brain to stay healthy.

Over the last fifty years the number of people living into their eighties and beyond has increased enormously. The main reason that symptoms of dementia have become more and more common is that there are more people around whose bodies are living longer so the declining health of their brains shows up dramatically.

Why do some functions decline as we age?

There are many answers to this question. First, on the level of evolution and natural selection, it's likely that mammals are not programmed to stay fit beyond their prime reproductive and child-rearing years. Specific, wholly natural, biological mechanisms appear to cause the brain to self-destruct. In fact, some parts of the brain appear to let themselves be destroyed without fighting back. Continuing research into specific mechanisms of brain destruction may reveal practical ways to manipulate or augment the brain's own self-repair and self-maintenance systems. The long-term benefit of this research, obviously, could contribute to our understanding of how to remain cognitively fit throughout life.

Vitamin E: Natural protection for your brain cells

Programmed cell death: brain-cell suicide

The mechanisms causing biological self-destruction of brain structures have attracted a lot of scientific and media attention recently. In some kinds of brain disease or injury, brain cells die because they produce self-destructive chemicals, or because they simply fail to take the necessary steps to keep themselves alive. In effect, they commit suicide. Some experiments have shown that the body gradually withdraws supportive, nutritive brain proteins called *growth factors* that normally sustain brain cells. As a result, the brain cells produce "killer proteins" that cause their own death. Brain-cell suicide can be delayed by increasing the supply of natural growth factors. Growth factor production can be increased by mental and physical exercise, surgical implants, and in some other ways that are discussed in the next chapter.

Free radicals: destructive brain-toxic chemicals

Highly reactive hydrogen, oxygen, and iron molecules with extra electrons, called free radicals, can be produced within the brain after brain injury. They also occur in a number of brain-based and brain-damaging disorders, such as chronic alcoholism, epilepsy, and AD. They kill brain cells by punching holes in the cell's protective membrane, releasing survival-essential substances and letting in toxins. Free radicals can be produced outside the brain by a wide variety of diseases and in response to lifestyle stres-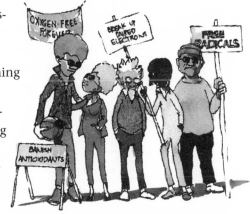

sors. Indeed, aging itself is believed to increase free radical production and lead to heightened oxidative brain-tissue damage.

Vitamin E: natural protection for your brain cells?
One of the best-known forms of protection against free radicals are *antioxidants*, also known as *free radical scavengers*. Vitamins C and E are both antioxidants. A variety of animal experiments over the past ten years have shown that vitamin E is effective in combating brain damage. In one experiment, rats given vitamin E injections after frontal lobe removal performed just as well on frontal-lobe-based intelligence tests as rats with undamaged frontal lobes. Other experiments have used rats whose carotid artery was blocked, which normally causes serious neuron loss and brain damage because it cuts off the supply of oxygen and fuel to the brain. These rats suffered little brain-cell loss if they were given vitamin E injections.

Vitamin E might therefore guard against brain-cell damage both by scavenging free radicals and by protecting the membranes that surround brain cells, thus combating a broad range of changes in the brain that occur in AD.

Although the experiments with rats mentioned above relied on injections or implanted pumps to get vitamin E into the brain — a procedure you obviously can't try at home — there are simpler ways of getting the brain-protecting benefit of this antioxidant. Other experiments have shown that dietary supplements can increase brain levels of vitamin E by 50 to 100 percent.

The question remains, however — does it do any good?

The research indicates that, at best, the benefit of vitamin E and other antioxidants is subtle. A widely cited report by the Alzheimer's Disease Cooperative Study, a consortium of Alzheimer's research centers sponsored by the U.S. National Institute on Aging, offered some evidence that vitamin E and another antioxidant called *selegiline* may help to delay the course of Alzheimer's among patients with the disease. Neither drug showed any effectiveness in improving symptoms, however. The NIA awarded the consortium $54 million in 2001 to perform further studies of a variety of drugs and supplements including vitamin E, but it is unlikely that antioxidants will provide any dramatic help to AD sufferers. Meanwhile, many doctors do recommend vitamin E supplements for older people with memory complaints, because it's an inexpensive, independently beneficial nutrient that, at the very least, will probably do no harm.

The current opinion about other antioxidants such as ginkgo and melatonin is similar. Extracts from the *ginkgo biloba tree*, which have been part of the Chinese pharmacopoeia for millennia, have been the subject of trials in Europe and North America that produced claims of beneficial effects on memory and alertness. The exact mechanism by which ginkgo might have any benefit is still a subject of investigation. Proponents have pointed to anti-clotting and antioxidant properties, and its ability to boost blood supply to the brain.

Like vitamin E, it is low-risk and non-invasive, so it is sometimes recommended to those with mild cognitive impairment or memory complaints.

Do painkillers help?

Some evidence has also been found for a possible protective effect of painkillers such as ibuprofen — collectively known as nonsteroidal anti-inflammatory drugs (NSAIDs) — perhaps by reducing the nerve cell inflammation that accompanies AD. As with the other supplements mentioned here, if NSAIDs do have any benefit, it probably lies in lowering the risk of developing Alzheimer's rather than reversing or slowing the disease once it has begun.

About estrogen

A few years ago, nearly 40 percent of postmenopausal American women had opted for hormone replacement therapy (HRT), a supplement of estrogen and progestin. The findings suggested that it protected them against osteoporosis, heart disease, and certain cancers, not to mention less life-threatening discomforts such as hot flashes and night sweats. The Women's Health Initiative recently undertook a large-scale study investigating the risks and benefits of estrogen/progestin supplements. An unexpected and distressing finding was that the hormone supplements actually seemed to increase rates of breast cancer, heart disease, and stroke.

A good study ended

That finding prompted the WHI to end the study prematurely. But the WHI is still studying the possible benefits of estrogen on the brain, based on other findings of a possible benefit of estrogen supplements in reducing the risk of AD. So far, independently of the WHI study, it looks like estrogen replacement therapy may lower Alzheimer's risk in women if it is begun relatively early, around the onset of menopause. It is probably not the case, based on available evidence, that estrogen supplements can affect the progression of AD once the disease has begun.

A large body of research since the mid-nineties into the connection between estrogen and Alzheimer's has pointed to several mechanisms by which this hormone may forestall dementia. It promotes the growth of dendrites — that is, helps brain cells to stay high-functioning by replacing lost connections between them. Estrogen also helps maintain the brain's *cholinergic system* in areas typically harmed by AD. The cholinergic system is the system that releases the neurotransmitter acetylcholine, crucial for proper attention and memory functions. Estrogen also appears to interact with growth factors to promote the survival and self-repair of neurons.

Given the more invasive nature of hormone supplements and recent findings suggesting that estrogen may do more harm than good when it comes to other diseases such as cancer, the use of estrogen to protect against dementia is more controversial than the use of vitamins, NSAIDs, ginkgo, or melatonin. Current indications are that if estrogen does have benefits, they may lie in a lower incidence of dementia after many years of taking the supplement starting at an age well before the risk of Alzheimer's onset.

Stress hormones: deadly to brain cells

Cortisol is a harmful, brain-toxic substance that is produced naturally by the body. It is one of a class of hormones released by the adrenal glands when the body is under stress. Cortisol reduces the blood-glucose energy supply to the brain, causing mental confusion and difficulties with short-term memory. It also interferes with the brain's neurotransmitters, crucial for proper communication from one brain cell to another. Eventually, high levels of cortisol resulting from chronic stress can kill brain cells by stimulating the production of free radicals. Chronically high levels of cortisol are bad under any circumstances, and they may play a role in raising the likelihood of dementia. Research has shown that high levels of cortisol are present in patients with AD.

One way the body can combat this harmful hormone is by reducing exposure to stress, and learning to control your response to stress. Relaxation techniques such as yoga, meditation, and biofeedback appear to help some people, as do enjoyable mental and social stimulation and physical exercise. Regular exercise also helps counteract brain degeneration because physically fit people tend to have a milder stress response, which, in turn, lowers cortisol levels. Aerobic exercise also boosts the supply of blood to the brain, which promotes mental clarity, and helps keep the cardiovascular system in good shape. Neurons draw on more energy when they are forced to become active. Increasing blood flow to the brain supplies the fuel neurons need on an ongoing basis.

Whether AD is a real or imagined threat the effort to dodge brain-harming substances is worth the extra attention. For those who now are struggling against AD, or for those who are caring for them, take heart. As you read this a great deal of serious, well-funded research into the causes and possible cures for AD in laboratory animals is beginning to translate into a few promising pharmaceutical products currently undergoing trials for practical application to the human condition. That is urgent work for the four million current sufferers and the epidemic coming when the baby boom enters old age.

References for Section 2
Diagnosing Alzheimer's:
Albert, M.S., et al. 2001. "Preclinical prediction of AD using neuro-psychological tests." *Journal of the International Neuropsychological Society* 7/5:631-9.

Johnson, K.A., et al. 1998. "Preclinical prediction of Alzheimer's disease using SPECT." *Neurology* 50/6:1563-71.

Killiany, R.J., et al. 2000. "Use of structural magnetic resonance imaging to predict who will get Alzheimer's disease." *Annals of Neurology* 47/4:430-9.

Wolf, H., et al. 2003. "A critical discussion of the role of neu-roimaging in mild cognitive impairment." *Acta Neurologica Scandinavica Supplementum* 179:52-76.

Alzheimer's and depression:
Hirono, N., et al. 1998. "Frontal lobe hypometabolism and depres-sion in Alzheimer's disease." *Neurology* 50/2:380-3.

Speck, C.E., et al. 1995. "History of depression as a risk factor for Alzheimer's disease." *Epidemiology* 6/4:366-9.

Weiner, M.F., S.D. Edland, and H. Luszczynska. 1994. "Prevalence and incidence of major depression in Alzheimer's disease." *American Journal of Psychiatry* 151/7:1006-9.

Effectiveness of vitamin E, ginkgo, melatonin, NSAIDs in protecting the brain:
Aisen, P.S., et al. 2003. "Effects of rofecoxib or naproxen vs. place-bo on Alzheimer disease progression: a randomized controlled trial." *JAMA* 289/21:2819-26.

Andrieu, S., et al. 2003. "Association of Alzheimer's disease onset with ginkgo biloba and other symptomatic cognitive treatments in a population of women aged 75 years and older from the EPI-DOS study." *Journals of Gerontology, Series A: Biological Sciences and Medical Sciences* 58/4:372-7.

Behan, W.M.H., et al. 1999. "Oxidative stress as a mechanism for quinolinic acid-induced hippocampal damage: protection by melatonin and deprynyl." *British Journal of Pharmacology* 128:1754-60.

Dongen. M., et al. 2003. "Ginkgo for elderly people with demen-tia and age-associated memory impairment: a randomized clinical trial." *Journal of Clinical Epidemiology* 56/4:367-76.

Gagne, B., et al. 2003. "Effects of estradiol, phytoestrogens, and ginkgo biloba extracts against 1-methyl-4-phenyl-pyridine-induced oxidative stress." *Endocrine* 1:89-96.

Grundman, M. 2000. "Vitamin E and Alzheimer's disease: the basis for additional clinical trials." *American Journal of Clinical Nutrition* 71 (Suppl.):630S-6S.

Grundman, M., and P. Delaney. 2002. "Antioxidant strategies for Alzheimer's disease." *Proceedings of the Nutrition Society* 61/2:191-202.

Inci, S., O.E. Ozcan, and K. Kilinc. 1998. "Time-level relationship for lipid peroxidation and the protective effect of alpha-tocopherol in experimental mild and severe brain injury." *Neurosurgery* 43/2:330-5.

Meydani, M., J.B. Macauley, and J.B. Blumberg. 1988. "Effect of dietary vitamin E and selenium on susceptibility of brain regions to lipid peroxidation." *Lipids* 23:405-9.

Monji A., et al. 1994. "Effect of dietary vitamin E on lipofuscin accumulation with age in the rat brain." *Brain Research* 634:62-8.

Sano, M., et al. 1997. "A controlled trial of selegiline, alpha-tocopherol, or both as treatment for Alzheimer's disease." *The New England Journal of Medicine* 336/17:1216-22.

Stephenson, J. 1996. "More evidence links NSAID, estrogen use with reduced Alzheimer risk." *JAMA* 275/18:1389-90.

Effects of estrogen on Alzheimer's risk:

Fillit, Howard M. 2002. "The role of hormone replacement therapy in the prevention of Alzheimer disease." *Archives of Internal Medicine* 162:1934-42.

Gagne, B., et al. 2003. "Effects of estradiol, phytoestrogens, and ginkgo biloba extracts against 1-methyl-4-phenyl-pyridine-induced oxidative stress." *Endocrine* 1:89-96.

Ghebremedhin, E., et al. 2001. "Gender and age modify the association between APOE and AD-related neuropathology." *Neurology* 56/12:1696-701.

Grodstein, F., T.B. Clarkson, and J.E. Manson. 2003. "Understanding the divergent data on postmenopausal hormone therapy." *The New England Journal of Medicine* 348/7:645-50.

Jacobs, D.M., et al. 1998. "Cognitive function in nondemented women who took estrogen after menopause." *Neurology* 50:368-73.

LeBlanc, Erin, et al. 2001. "Hormone replacement therapy and cognition: systematic review and meta-analysis." *JAMA* 285/11:1489-99.

Manly, J.J., et al. 2000. "Endogenous estrogen levels and Alzheimer's disease among postmenopausal women." *Neurology* 54:833-7.

Mulnard, R.A., et al. 2000. "Estrogen replacement therapy for treatment of mild to moderate Alzheimer disease: a randomized controlled trial." Alzheimer's Disease Cooperative Study. *JAMA* 283/8:1007-15.

Thal, L.J., et al. 2003. "Estrogen levels do not correlate with improvement in cognition." *Archives of Neurology* 60/2:209-12.

Women's Health Initiative. 2002. "Risks and benefits of estrogen plus progestin in healthy postmenopausal women: principal results from the Women's Health Initiative randomized controlled trial." *JAMA* 288/3:321-33.

Zandi, P.P., et al. 2002. "Hormone replacement therapy and incidence of Alzheimer disease in older women: the Cache County Study." *JAMA* 288/17:2123-9.

Effectiveness of cholinesterase inhibitors for treating Alzheimer's:

Francis, P.T., et al. 1999. "The cholinergic hypothesis of Alzheimer's disease: a review of progress." *Journal of Neurology, Neurosurgery, and Psychiatry* 66/2:137-47.

Lilienfeld, S. 2003. "Cholinesterase inhibitors for Alzheimer disease." *JAMA* 289/18:2360.

Trinh, N.H., et al. 2003. "Efficacy of cholinesterase inhibitors in the treatment of neuropsychiatric symptoms and functional impairment in Alzheimer disease: a meta-analysis." *JAMA* 289/2:210-16.

Alzheimer's vaccine:

Nicoll, J.A.R., et al. 2003. "Neuropathology of Alzheimer's disease after immunization with amyloid-ß peptide: a case report." *Nature Medicine* 9/4:448-52.

Schenk, D., et al. 1999. "Immunization with amyloid-beta attenuates Alzheimer-disease-like pathology in the PDAPP mouse." *Nature* 400:173-7.

Neurotrophins (growth factors):

Deckwerth, T.L., and E.M. Johnson Jr. 1993. "Temporal analysis of events associated with programmed cell death (apoptosis) of sympathetic neurons deprived of nerve growth factor." *Journal of Cell Biology* 123/5:1207-22.

Frade , J.M., and Y.A. Barde. 1998. "Nerve growth factor: two receptors, multiple functions." *Bioessays* 20/2: 137-45.

Rich, K.M. 1992. "Neuronal death after trophic factor deprivation." *Journal of Neurotrauma* 9 (Suppl. 1):S61-9.

Russo-Neustadt, A. 2003. "Brain-derived neurotrophic factor, behavior, and new directions for the treatment of mental disorders." *Seminars in Clinical Neuropsychiatry* 8/2:109-18.

Tatebayashi, Y., et al. 2003. "The dentate gyrus neurogenesis: a therapeutic target for Alzheimer's disease." *Acta neuropathologica* 105/3:225-32.

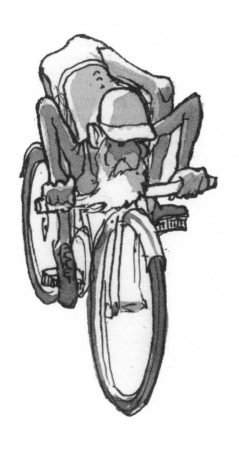

PREVENTING AND REVERSING COGNITIVE DECLINE WITH AGE BASED ON CURRENT RESEARCH RESULTS

OUTMODED BELIEFS ABOUT THE BRAIN

NEW FINDINGS

PRACTICAL WAYS TO APPLY
SCIENTIFICALLY PROVEN RESEARCH

HOPE FOR THE FUTURE FROM THE
BRAIN'S OWN HEALING SYSTEMS

Outmoded Beliefs About the Brain

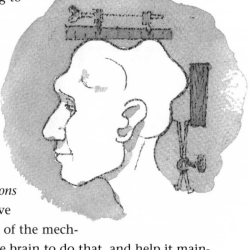

Very little of what you're going to read in this chapter could have been written a mere ten years ago. We now know that adult brains, even old brains, retain their power to replenish their supply of *neurons* (brain cells). We have learned about some of the mechanisms that help the brain to do that, and help it maintain the health of cells it already has. We can't control or replicate the brain, but we can encourage the brain to apply its enormous resources to the job of taking care of itself.

The adult human body can grow new cells in its brain

Until very recently psychology textbooks said "in the adult brain, nervous pathways are fixed and immutable; everything may die, nothing may be regenerated." This pessimistic view, put forward by Nobel Prize-winning Spanish neuroscientist Ramon y Cajal over sixty years ago, has discouraged interest in developing drugs, treatments, and therapies for brain-damaging injuries as well as for common age-related cognitive decline.

Certain parts of the brain specialize in a specific skill but other areas can take over if forced to

Luckily, we now have proof that any mental ability or function — language, memory, motivation — are not housed exclusively in a specific part of the brain. Back in the nineteenth century, when practitioners of the pseudoscience of phrenology claimed to be able to gauge a person's intelligence and even moral rectitude by "reading" the bumps and contours on the skull, they imagined that the bumps were shaped by the brain beneath. The faulty assumption behind this belief is still with us, and leads us to overemphasize the degree to which specific brain functions are localized in specific areas. In reports of experiments, even using sophisticated imaging technology invented only about fifteen years ago, such as PET or fMRI, researchers sometimes simplify complex, widespread patterns of brain activation in their search for the brain region underlying a skill such as reading, or a disability such as dyslexia.

In the brain, redundancy is good

The most dramatic kinds of evidence come from a surgical operation called a *hemispherectomy* that removes the entire cortex on one side of the brain in order to correct severe epileptic seizures. Each *hemisphere* (side) specializes in some way. The right hemisphere processes visual forms in space used in designing structures or having a good sense of direction. Males are more specialized that way than females. Most language skills are processed on the left side. Even if the left hemisphere is removed, which destroys the dominant language regions of the brain, a young patient will recover full language ability within a relatively short period of time.

The explanation is that regions of the right hemisphere are able to help with some language skills. These areas only become fully activated if the left-brain regions are destroyed.

Why stroke-therapy works when the patient works
Even though this kind of redundancy and flexibility is most pronounced in children, it's never completely lost. This same kind of imaging technology reveals that many brain regions reorganize themselves after an adult suffers a brain injury such as a stroke. That take-over ability engages only when the brain is forced to use that skill. Stroke patients who work the hardest during rehabilitation tend to regain more of their lost skills. Very recent advances in brain research are making it increasingly clear that the adult human brain has built-in mechanisms for adjusting to and compensating for brain injury.

New Findings

How to keep your brain cells healthy: "use it or lose it" vs. "wear and tear"

We are beginning to understand some of the specific cellular and chemical mechanisms by which using the brain serves to maintain it.

But it seems like the brain might just wear out gradually like a car engine

By the "wear and tear" model, we mean the idea that what happens as you get older is that your brain cells, like certain other parts of your body or like the brake pads on your car, gradually get worn down by use. If that wear and tear theory is what actually happens, then the less you push your brain the longer it will last. Of course, you have to protect it, not wreck it, and maintain it regularly like changing the oil. In some ways that is right.

There's evidence that ordinary by-products of cell metabolism, such as what are called free radicals (see page 79), can damage neurons. (For example, they cause damage by harming the cells' ability to maintain themselves or create new connections.) Certain "stress" hormones known as glucocorticoids, naturally produced in the body, have also been shown to interfere with memory function and even kill neurons when their levels are consistently high. Even high levels of oxygen can damage brain cells. Perhaps, then, our brains slow down as we age simply as the result of a wearing away of brain cells, or a decreased ability of neurons to respond to new challenges, because the very fact of living exposes our brain cells to toxins. So no matter what we do, sooner or later cells wear out or die and force us into senility the way the inevitable erosion of cartilage in a catcher's knee forces him to retire from baseball by the time he reaches his mid-thirties? Wrong!

Why mental exercise conditions the brain to perform better longer

What the "wear and tear" assumptions ignore is the fact that brain cells have self-support and regeneration mechanisms that are actually stimulated by use. The use of neurons may protect them. This "exercise" effect early in childhood and adult life can also help avoid brain degeneration with age. Active mental exercise boosts genetically triggered repair mechanisms that enable the cells to maintain themselves and grow. Mental effort may also trigger the production of the brain's own natural antioxidants. The "use it or lose it" principle may in fact provide a better explanation for the effect of glucocorticoids on stress response than the "wear and tear" model, because excess glucocorticoids impede the fuel uptake of cells, thereby interfering with their proper function. With Alzheimer's, for example, it isn't increased activity of certain brain regions, but *decreased* activity. Alzheimer's-diseased brains show a reduction in the products of genetically-triggered repair, and the brain areas affected show decreased metabolism.

A brain cell is like a telephone: there's no use having it unless it's wired up

Consider that a brain cell doesn't do any good unless it's connected to other brain cells so that it can send and receive information. During the early years of life, and even before that in the womb humans have more neurons than they ever will again. From birth to puberty our superabundant brain cells are getting winnowed down through a cutthroat competition for connections. If a cell fails to establish a connection, or enough connections with enough other cells, or if already-existing connections aren't used, it dies.

What determines whether connections are made?

It's partly just a matter of some cells being defective in the first place, much as many of the sperm cells produced by a healthy adult male are defective and nonfunctional. It's also partly due to genetic preprogramming. But it's more decided by which ones are needed.

Evaluation has given humans a special survival advantage over other animals

Instead of imposing a fixed blueprint for all the 100 trillion or so connections between neurons, our brain comes laid out with the main "cable highways" and leaves the fine wiring to be determined by trial and error. A rat's whiskers are essential to navigating in the dark. If a newborn rat has its whiskers trimmed, the part of the cortex of its brain that decodes the whiskers' sensory input changes. The connections which had been set up by the rat's genetic blueprint whither away, instead of developing complex branches.

97

Getting into plastics

Quick, in what movie was Dustin Hoffman told to get into plastics? A human's ability to create and change new brain circuits all its life is called "plasticity." Plasticity can also be seen in the tiny protrusions on the neurons called *spines* and *filopodia*. These microscopic structures expand and contract on a minute-by-minute basis in response to sensory input. They work on a "use it or lose it" principle — if the input crossing a given synapse isn't enough, it's pruned away.

Recruiting the troops

A very recent experiment with newborn ferrets shows that new experiences after birth can even cause an entire section of the brain to be recruited to perform a different function from the one normally housed there. Ferrets, of course, can see and hear, and have different kinds of brain cells, in different regions of the cortex, specialized for each of these skills. When experimenters prevent the nerve-carrying sounds from reaching the brain, the part of a ferret's brain that usually interprets sounds switches over to handling visual input, and develops specialized vision cells normally present only in the visual cortex. Then, the ferrets literally see with their auditory cortex. This reorganization seems to be essentially the same kind that occurs in humans — even adults — who lose one of their senses by a stroke, for example.

In the brain, quality is more important than quantity

Brain cells that get exercise develop better and thicker insulation (called *myelin*) around their *axon* (a long branch that transmits information to other cells). The *dendrites* (shorter fingers that receive information from other cells) multiply their branches. Growth of neurons in this way increases the brain's size and weight all the way through mid-adolescence. This also means that, even though many cells and synapses have been weeded out by that age, those that remain are better developed and more efficient and effective for the skills and knowledge that have been acquired. The take-home message is this: the quantity of brain cells counts less than their quality — and the evidence suggests that high-quality brain cells are developed by using them.

"As the twig is bent, so grows the tree"
Childhood is a particularly crucial "use it or lose it" time. Some aspects of language and vision, for example, develop during critical periods that will close for good if those skills don't develop by the right age. (For details see *Learn Faster & Remember More* by the same authors.) Many skills are laid down early. Nearly all Olympic athletes started their sport before the time they were seven. Once you learn how to ride a bike, you never really forget. Though your reflexes may slow down, you never have to go back to training wheels. Adults can learn new skills later in life, of course, but in youth neural pathways easily begin to get laid down that can enrich an entire life.

Any skills, if learned and used early in life, may become so strongly wired into permanent circuitry that they can function effortlessly thereafter.

What about adult brain conditioning? Too late?
Introducing enriched cognitive routines establish and maintain skills throughout life. Animal experiments have established repeatedly that laboratory rats weaned

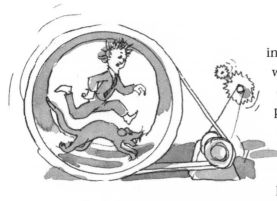

in an environment without play activities can catch up to the performance level of enriched-environment rats in solving spatial problems, once they're given the same richness of exposure. Other studies have shown that a bird's hippocampus — a seat of spatial memory — will grow when the bird is given food hiding-and-retrieving tasks well on in life, even if it was denied that experience when young.

Mature brains grow and lose connections constantly depending on whether they are needed

Even old lab rats grow bigger and better brains when placed in a varied, challenging, socially rich environment. Their dendritic branches proliferate or die back depending on their friends and toys. The outreaching "fingers" on their cells (*dendrites*) grow "spines" (the tiny contact points between cells), which are amazingly sensitive to mental challenges or inactivity.

The human brain isn't a static object after childhood, like a block of stone slowly worn down or chipped away with time; it's a collection of trillions of pieces — dendrites, spines, and *synapses* (connecting points) — that are in a constant state of flux and are constantly changing their size and shape as they are asked to interact with the world around them

Until five years ago they said "the mature human brain could never grow brand new cells"

Fatter neurons are only one reason that brains can get

bigger and better late in life. Two bodies of independent research (the Salk Institute in San Diego and Princeton University) reported in March 1999 new evidence that adult lab animals were growing new brain cells. A Purdue researcher, Joseph Altman, actually offered evidence for this thirty-five years ago, but most scientists simply dismissed his findings at the time.

In the Salk study, mice that exercised regularly on a running wheel grew twice as many new brain cells as other mice. The new cells appeared in the hippocampus, a part of the brain crucial for memory and learning. A confirming study (Elizabeth Gould of Princeton) found that challenging mental tasks on a sustained program not only spurred the production of new hippocampal brain cells, but helped maintain existing ones as well. As Gould herself put it, "It's a classic case of 'use it or lose it'."

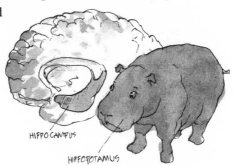

HIPPOCAMPUS

HIPPOPOTAMUS

Practical Ways to Apply Scientifically Proven Research

A Swedish-American team led by the Salk Institute's Fred Gage recently confirmed that, in fact, adult human brains can and do grow new neurons throughout life.

Scientists learn about how the human brain operates in a variety of ways. An increasingly sophisticated arsenal of scanning techniques is becoming available to get inside a living, functioning brain without causing any harm. These brain-scanning methods include CAT, PET, fMRI, and SPECT. Dissecting the brains of people who elected to donate their organs to science after death can show up differences in the brain's anatomy and physiology in people with and without Alzheimer's (AD) for example.

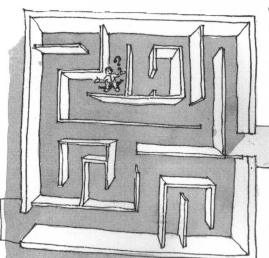

What autopsies of Alzheimer's patients' brains have shown AD appears as structural changes (plaques and tangles) among the neurons in certain parts of the *cortex* (the brain's outer layer) and hippocampus. As brain cells atrophy in those areas, those parts of the brain shrink. The brain has a protective layer inside does. Its size reveals the high-water mark of brain size in that individual's life. The less that layer has expanded outward the greater the likelihood of contracting AD. Bigger is better. Those who have built up a "functional reserve" of well-developed brain cells have a kind of built-in protection against AD. It may also explain why some people develop the characteristic structural signs of AD without showing any signs of cognitive impairment.

Even an inherited brain disease is blocked by mental exercise
Some other degenerative diseases that affect the brain are more strongly genetically determined than AD. Huntington's disease, for example — the disorder that felled songwriter Woody Guthrie — is caused by a dominant gene that is inherited 50 percent of the time by the offspring of someone with the disease. In other words, if the son or daughter of someone with Huntington's lives long enough, chances are fifty-fifty they will get it too — regardless of their general health, habits, or lifestyle. And if one of a pair of identical twins has Huntington's, chances are 100 percent that the twin sibling will get it.

On the other hand, one of the twins can show more severe symptoms at a younger age than the other, and deteriorate more rapidly. This indicates that even with a genetically caused neurological disease, the course of progression of the disease can be influenced by the environment.

A very recent experiment by a team of Oxford researchers shows how a mentally challenging environment can reduce the bad effects of a Huntington's-like disorder in mice. The researchers raised half of a group of mice with a Huntington's-type gene in standard cages, and half in "environmentally enriched" cages filled with a constantly-rotating collection of toys and games. Week by week, all the mice were tested on two separate tasks designed to reveal symptoms of the disease. The "standard-environment" mice showed symptoms earlier than "enriched-environment" mice in both tasks. In one task, only about half of the "enriched" mice had developed symptoms by the end of the experiment, while 100 percent of the "standard" mice had. In the other task, only one of fifteen enriched mice showed symptoms by the end of the period compared, again, to 100 percent of the "standard" Huntington's mice.

A good education, formal or self-taught, helps protect against AD

Many studies have pointed to the conclusion that people with higher education and more challenging occupations are less likely to get AD. In fact, one statistical analysis of the results of several of these studies came to the conclusion that educational level is a stronger predictor of the likelihood of developing AD than any of the commonly-cited factors, including family history.

The problem, though, is that a correlation does not necessarily prove a cause. Educational level and occupation cluster with other lifestyle factors — exercise, diet, interests, consumption of alcohol and nicotine — that have an impact on many diseases, including dementia. That's why researchers always seek to control for additional factors by keeping them constant. One way to do this is to study only people who have the same lifestyle but different levels of education, or different occupations, and see who develops AD and who doesn't.

A case study: The smart sisters who never got AD
A careful study of nuns launched in 1991 followed the cognitive health of 678 members of the School Sisters of Notre Dame congregation born before 1917. It was an ideal sampling of people with largely similar lifestyle variables. Several subsequent studies have drawn on carefully selected subgroups within the entire nun pool to investigate possible correlations between dementia and other factors that vary among the participants. All the participating nuns agreed in advance to allow their brains to be analyzed after death, so researchers have been able not only to test their cognitive function on an annual basis, but to identify structural signs of AD at autopsy.

The education factor
One study that drew on the Nun Study data examined correlations between level of education and cognitive function among a subset of 247 of the nuns. These nuns were carefully chosen for similar lifestyles, but differences in educational level. Remarkably, despite the equivalence in adult lifestyle, highly educated nuns were twice as likely to avoid Alzheimer's and other dementias late in life than less educated nuns. This offers some proof that the "protective" effect of educa-

High Idea Density and Grammatical Complexity in Writing Style: A Sign of Low Risk for AD?

"Idea density" is a measure of the average number of "ideas" per ten words. "Grammatical complexity" is graded according to how much embedding and syntactic subordination a sentence shows. Here is an excerpt comparing the nun who scored lowest in idea density and grammatical complexity (below left) with the nun who scored highest (below right). These are from autobiographical essays the nuns wrote when they were in their early twenties.

The sister who wrote the sample on the left died with AD, while the one who wrote the sentence on the right was (at the time of the study) still alive with no cognitive impairment.

I was born in Eau Claire, Wis, on May 24, 1913 and was baptized in St James Church.

The happiest day of my life so far was my First Communion Day which was in June nineteen hundred and twenty when I was but eight years of age, and four years later in the same month I was confirmed by Bishop D.D. McGavick.

The researchers computed an idea density score of 3.9 and a grammatical complexity rating of 0 for the sentence excerpt on the left. The low grammatical complexity score reflects a simple one-clause sentence with no embedding. Here is how the idea density score was computed:

Idea 1: I was born
Idea 2: born in Eau Claire, Wis
Idea 3: born on May 24, 1913
Idea 4: I was baptized
Idea 5: was baptized in church
Idea 6: I was baptized in St. James Church
Idea 7: I was born and was baptized

Assuming 18 "words," seven ideas divided by 18 = 3.9. The sentence on the right was given an idea density score of 8.6, and a grammatical complexity rating of 7.

Sentences high in grammatical complexity impose more demands on working memory than ones low in grammatical complexity. A writing style high in grammatical complexity may reflect speech habits that impose frequent demands to exercise working memory skills.

To see how taxing embedding and subordination can be, try deciphering the made-up example below. This kind of sentence is in fact so difficult to decipher that, even though it does not violate any formal rules of grammar, any editor could rewrite it:

The fact that the kid told you about that I don't like you bothers me a lot.

(Rewrite: It bothers me a lot that the kid told you about the fact that I don't like you.)

tion early in life is not simply due to other lifestyle factors — diet, marriage status, occupation, or what have you — correlating with education level.

The complexity of thought factor, at a young age
Even more striking findings were obtained in an investigation of the relation between writing style in early adult life and development of Alzheimer's in old age among a subset of ninety-three nuns. All ninety-three participants had submitted short autobiographies written after their religious training and before taking their vows, typically when they were in their early twenties. The authors of this study analyzed those early writing

samples for "idea density" and "grammatical complexity" (see box, page 106). Those nuns who had written samples scoring low in these respects were more likely to have low cognitive test scores late in life, with low idea density showing a stronger association with poor late-life cognitive performance than low grammatical complexity. The most striking finding, though, was that all those nuns with low idea density early in life developed AD in old age, while not a single one with high idea density did so.

Why would a high education and a relatively sophisticated writing style early in life tend to prevent serious dementias in old age?
One interpretation of the findings in the research with nuns (see A case study: the smart sisters . . . , page 105) is that experiences and habits from childhood to early adulthood help to build up a "cognitive reserve" or "brain reserve capacity" that can be drawn on later in life. That is, extra, more richly developed neural pathways laid down early in life can give the aging brain more of a reserve to draw on, even if some neurons die or become less efficient.

The mental exercise approach to protecting against AD
Another theory — perfectly compatible with the mental complexity findings — holds that at least some of the protective effect of education and "idea density" is brought about by constant mental exercise that keeps neurons alive and healthy. In fact, education helps lay the groundwork for lifelong patterns of intellectually challenging activities, and "idea density" in young-adult writing style tends to predict lasting habits of processing

complex linguistic structures. Just as physical exercise boosts the flow of blood and oxygen to the body as a whole, mental exercise increases the supply of blood-borne nutrients to the brain. This in turn helps ward off the brain-toxic effects of the glucocorticoid "stress" hormone and may also serve to protect against free radicals (see Common Substances That May Harm the Brain, page 78). What's more, increased brain work stimulates DNA repair of damaged brain cells.

Proof that education trumps brain disease
Support for the role of the protective effect of education against AD also comes from brain-scan studies. For example, among patients with equivalent degrees of disease severity, blood flow to damaged regions of the brain is lower in patients with more advanced education. Given that reduced blood flow is a physical symptom of AD, this means that, on a *physical* level, the well-educated patients had a measurably more severe AD than the others — and yet, in their *cognitive* ability they showed no more signs of the disease than the poorly-educated patients whose brain scans showed less severe symptoms. So it may be that structural effects of AD in the brain — plaques and tangles, neuron loss, reduced blood flow — may be partially overcome by a greater reserve of neurons, synapses, and pathways built up over a lifetime of mental stimulation.

Evidence that lifelong patterns of stimulating activities and interests may be as important as early education
Evidence of forestalling dementia comes from studies that show a strong relationship between occupation and risk of dementia. An influential French study

showed that the risk of dementia among laborers in Bordeaux is two to three times greater than among professionals. Occupational status is in fact a far more important variable than education alone. The preventive effect of varied and mentally challenging occupations on AD has been confirmed in many other studies in the last decade, in the United States, Italy, and Israel.

It may seem that such findings about correlations between education or occupation and brain health are not very useful. After all, once you're 50 or 60, you can't do anything about the fact that you decided not to go to law school thirty or forty years ago. Nor can you go back in time to choose a more stimulating career. So what good does it do you to know about that research?

Discoveries about the role that education or career choices may play in keeping your brain healthy are just part of a pattern that is emerging from a broader range of studies.

Activities that you choose for yourself throughout life, including in old age, can help to preserve the health of your brain
One study reported recently in the *New England Journal of Medicine* observed a group of 469 subjects aged 75 or older for a period of several years. The researchers were particularly interested in testing the claim that participation in certain types of leisure activities might lower the risk of dementia. All of the subjects were tested and found to be free of dementia at the start of the study.

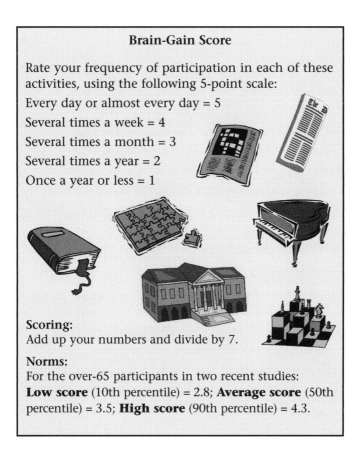

Brain-Gain Score

Rate your frequency of participation in each of these activities, using the following 5-point scale:

Every day or almost every day = 5

Several times a week = 4

Several times a month = 3

Several times a year = 2

Once a year or less = 1

Scoring:
Add up your numbers and divide by 7.

Norms:
For the over-65 participants in two recent studies:
Low score (10th percentile) = 2.8; **Average score** (50th percentile) = 3.5; **High score** (90th percentile) = 4.3.

Over a period of a little over five years, about a quarter of the subjects in the group developed dementia. After adjusting for age, sex, education, other medical illness, and cognitive test performance at the start of the study, the researchers found that reading, playing board games, playing a musical instrument, and dancing were associated with a reduced risk of dementia.

Two other recent studies by researchers at the Alzheimer's Disease Center in Chicago led to the same conclusion: The more cognitively stimulating activities older people pursued on a regular basis, the less likely they were to develop dementia. In plain terms, those researchers found that if you were over 65 and raised your activity level from the 10th percentile (i.e., 90 percent of your age-mates are more active than you) to the 90th percentile (you're more active than 90 percent of your age-mates), you could cut your Alzheimer's risk in half. That rise in activity level could be achieved just by increasing your frequency of doing such things as solving puzzles, playing board games, and going to museums from several times a month to several times a week. (See Brain-Gain Score, page 111.)

You don't need to study for a Ph.D. in nuclear physics to benefit from a more mentally active lifestyle
The activities in question are easily within anyone's capabilities. They're not hard or unpleasant, and they're not necessarily the kinds of things you'd think you needed to do to exercise your brain. (See Section 4) Indeed, most activities found to reduce risk of dementia also involve social interaction as well as engaging mental activity. Far from being unpleasant hard work, these activities are fun.

Most people are more concerned about their memory than about their prowess in games like charades. But pantomime games like charades are actually sensitive tests of dementia, and are more revealing of cognitive decline than memory tests in an important sense. While healthy elderly people tend to have relatively accurate perceptions of their own memory skills, they tend to overestimate their performance on a number of other less IQ-like skills, such as the skills involved in pantomime games. In that sense, charades can tell them more that they don't already know about the state of their brain than memory tests can.

In addition to the workout that games of charades can give to cognitive skills, they also serve as an excuse for social interaction, and even provide a little of physical exercise. All those factors — mental, social, and physical stimulation — have been shown to help the brain stay fit and healthy.

What a lively mind looks like in the brain

Researchers Jacobs, Schall, and Scheibel have discovered what the protective effects of an enriched life look like. The first branching split of a dendrite is called "first-order," the second level "second-order," and so on. In postmortem analyses of Wernicke's area (a part of the brain used in language), they found that the higher the educational level, the more higher-level branching (fourth-level and above) there was in that part of that person's brain.

One of the most important proofs that application of the "use it or lose it" concept leads to successful aging is a study of over 5,000 adults who were tested over a period of up to thirty-five years. The results point to several variables that may lower the risk of cognitive decline in old age. One cluster of factors includes above-average education and occupations involving work that is high in complexity and low in routine. Another cluster of factors includes interesting hobbies and leisure pursuits that involve complex and intellectually stimulating environments, such as extensive reading, travel, going to cultural events, pursuing continuing education, and participation in clubs and professional associations

Your brain is not so much like the knees of a baseball catcher as like the heart of a runner

Yes, exercise accelerates your heart rate and, on the theory that every heart has a preset number of beats before it wears out, might be thought to get you more quickly to your death. But that's not the way it really works. Using your heart strengthens it, lengthens its life, and improves the overall quality of life of the body that houses it. All the current evidence from experimental studies is showing that this is the way our brains work as well. It pays big dividends to make a constant effort to keep brains active and challenged, in order to keep them as healthy as a runner keeps his or her heart.

How to enrich your environment: Curiosity doesn't kill the cat, it makes the cat smarter
The idea that novelty helps the brain stay young and limber is true.

If you encounter a novel situation, your brain starts to figure out what's going on and what (if anything) to do about it. "What's happening here?" means basically "how does this relate to other situations I've been in?"; "what can I do about it?" means "which tools from my cognitive toolbox should I pull out and use?"

In any new situation you're challenged to find meaning by relating something new to something old. What's old is, of course, already accessible in a well-organized form in your brain. Somehow, your brain has to figure out how to handle the process of relating one thing to another in order to understand the new things that it's faced with.

Our language is filled with examples. When a politician talks about the "health" of the economy, or about what sort of fiscal "remedy" might "cure" what "ails" it, he's invoking something solid and familiar (the health of your body) in order to talk about something relatively abstract (the economy). That kind of analogy can serve as a useful bridge from something you do understand to something you don't.

Three crucial steps in brain activity
First, there's the new situation. Second, there's the trick of relating the new situation to something familiar. Third, there's the store of knowledge about familiar things to draw on when you try to understand something new.

Common sense says that greater age means, if anything, a larger store of knowledge to work with. Common sense also says, though, that people are less likely to put themselves in novel situations the older they get — both because more things are familiar (and, conversely, fewer things are novel) and because people tend to become set in their ways. When that happens the mental exercise of relating new to old will tend to decline steadily with increasing age.

New things tend to tax crucial working memory skills more than old ones. A simple example: When you get a number from directory assistance and you don't have a pen handy, you have to use your working memory to hold a phone number in your head long enough to dial it. But if you already know the number, all you have to keep in mind is the person you're calling, which automatically triggers access to the number in your long-term memory.

So until you've made sense of a novel situation, you're going to have to rely on a crucial, short-term memory system that has a tendency to weaken with age. The process of relating this new thing to that familiar one also draws on prefrontal brain regions that older people tend to tap less often. They need to put more effort into learning new things and coping with unfamiliar situations. But it also means that the more novelty they choose to deal with, the more likely they are to preserve faculties they'll need in order to stay mentally young and healthy.

You can't build yourself a better brain, or maintain what you already have, unless you want to. A janitor in the Library of Congress doesn't acquire an encyclopedic knowledge merely by being in the presence of so many books. You need to explore and interact with the learning resources that are available to you, which will have a positive effect on the health of your brain. Section 4 of this book provides eighty-seven original, brain-training exercises designed to sharpen the six most crucial mental skills.

A Case Study: The Smarter Cat

Over 30 years ago, Richard Held made a point that is still crucially important for those of us interested in "optimal aging." He designed an ingenious experiment which looked at how the visual system of the cat develops. The experiment showed that only certain sorts of environmental stimulation will lead to the development of more acute visual processing centers in kittens' brains. The critical point of the experiment was that proper development only happens when the stimulation results from active exploration, as opposed to purely passive exposure. The two kittens were linked by a carousel-like contraption that allowed one kitten to explore freely while the other could not. Every time the active kitten moved towards an interesting visual stimulus, the passive one would be automatically swiveled towards an equivalent object or image. In this way, both kittens were exposed to the same visual environment, but only one did so in an active manner. When the brains of the cats were eventually examined, only the cat who had explored the environment actively had developed superior visual processing abilities.

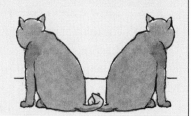

HOPE FOR THE FUTURE FROM THE BRAIN'S OWN HEALING SYSTEMS

What you should know about stem cells and growth factors.

An exciting but controversial, new avenue of treatment for brain diseases comes from recent experiments with stem cells. These are general-purpose cells that can divide and differentiate to produce specialist cells, including brain cells. Some scientists see stem cells as a source of treatment for brain damage and degenerative brain diseases.

How a stem cell works

When a human egg is first fertilized by a sperm, it becomes a single cell from which all cells of the body-to-be will be created. This "mother of all stem cells" is what biologists call *totipotent,* meaning that it has unlimited creative capacity. One level down from the totipotent "mother" stem cell are *pluripotent* cells, capable of generating all the cells of the body but not the placenta that the fetus needs to survive. By a process of division and specialization, further levels of stem cells are created, leading ultimately to each particular cell — blood, brain, skin, etc. — of the body.

Some of the more specialized stem cells continue to exist in the body after birth, all life long. Blood stem cells, for example, generate new red blood cells, white blood cells, and platelets until death. They can't generate all the types of cells in the human body but they're still capable of generating a number of important specific cells of a general type.

Good news: Adult human brains do have stem cells
Until very recently, the accepted wisdom has been that humans carry no stem cells for the brain into adulthood because central nervous system cells in the brain and spine can't regenerate the way that the cells in the skin, blood, and other body systems do. As with so much other long-accepted knowledge about the brain, this postulate turns out to be wrong.

A chemical called bromodeoxyuredine (BrdU) is used as a kind of marker to pinpoint rapid cell division, as happens most dramatically when healthy cells turn cancerous. In 1998, Fred Gage of the Salk Institute performed autopsies on several terminal cancer patients who had been injected with the chemical before they died. The presence of BrdU in their brains showed that their brain cells had been dividing and generating new brain cells. Other studies since then have shown such *neurogenesis* (the ongoing regeneration of neurons) in the brains of adult animals, including primates closely related to humans. Recently, a group of researchers at Sweden's Karolinska Institute demonstrated that the adult human brain carries stem cells as well.

Why research on stem cells in the human brain started to explode only months after researchers discovered them in the brain
Stem cells reside quietly near the brain ventricles (fluid-filled structures in the brain's interior) until spurred into action by growth factors. They can then develop

into either of the two most general classes of brain cell, neurons or *glial cells*. (Glial cells are a special type of cell that researchers have only recently come to treat with the respect they deserve; formerly thought to provide little more than a structural "glue" for neurons, it turns out they manufacture and store substances essential to the survival and health of the neurons.)

When someone suffers a stroke or other brain injury, the stem cells are switched from their usual resting state into the production of specialized brain cells that migrate to the injury site. And most bizarrely of all, when brain stem cells are taken from mice and injected into the tails of other mice, they develop into blood cells! The mechanism for this effect isn't clear, but there must be something in that part of the mouse's body — specific growth factors, perhaps — that can move even a stem cell from a different body system into becoming a blood cell. Suffice it to say that brain stem cells are still somewhat mysterious, but clearly have tremendous potential for brain maintenance and repair. They're like money in the savings account of a retiree, spent only in small amounts except in case of emergency. It would be nice, of course, to figure out how to have more of those precious funds to draw on.

Hi-tech ways to boost brain stem cell activity
One of the most controversial aspects of stem cell research has to do with harvesting the type of stem cells from aborted human fetuses that can grow into any type of cell the body may need. The hope is that such cells may be coaxed into generating any of a number of kinds of more specialized cells, and then implanted into the body or brain of a person with a

disease of a corresponding cell or organ type, such as diabetes (pancreatic cells), heart disease (heart cells), or Parkinson's or Alzheimer's (brain cells). This "coaxing" is a matter of switching on the right genes in the stem cell that trigger development into just the right kind of more specialized cell. Recent evidence indicates that this result may be accomplished by identifying the appropriate growth factor (see page 122) that spurs the cell in the desired direction. An even simpler technique would be to extract fetal tissue that has already become specialized in the right direction. This kind of experiment has in fact already been successfully performed by a Swedish team led by Anders Bjorklund, who implanted fetal brain cells into the brains of Parkinson's patients.

Further research now shows that a patient's own stem cells can be manipulated to generate brain cells of the right type, an approach that avoids the politically and socially controversial issue of harvesting fetal tissue. It also avoids the medically critical problems when implants are rejected by the recipient's immune system.

Just don't forget to use your brain

It's important to remember, though, that even with a procedure as invasive as fetal implants, the "use it or lose it" doctrine still applies — just as it does to newborns. In other words, if implanted cells are not used for the purpose for which they're implanted, they'll die. A well-functioning mind develops out of an intricate interplay between biological endowment and life experience. An infant given all the brain cells in the universe won't develop a good mind unless those neurons are linked up and enlarged through an active exploration of the environment. The same principle applies, as well, to an adult recipient of stem cells. In animal models, when implants are combined with a program of mental stimulation, they stand a much better chance of success than the implants alone.

The upshot of the profusion of advice and research findings reported on a daily basis in the medical journals and the media is that many factors influence healthy brain development and aging, and you can't expect to find a single magic bullet. But no matter what, brain-cell development, maintenance, and repair are guided by the uses to which we put our minds, both in childhood or adulthood.

The brain's own miracle cure: nerve growth factors
"Fine," you're thinking. "You've told me about lots of fancy research and given me some advice about keeping my brain healthy in the long run. But I want something that will automatically make my brain work better right away. Something that will help my neurons stay sharp, just like when I was twenty-five. Like ginkgo, but more powerful."

All right, there is such a thing. We can't sell it to you, but we do know where you can get it. It's actually never been approved by the FDA, so you can't get it from your doctor, but it's legal. And we can guarantee that it'll blow ginkgo out of the water.

What is this miracle drug? There are actually a few versions of it, and they have long, technical-sounding names, so you'll have to bear with us a minute. Here are a few of them: BDNF, IGF-I, and NT3, 4, and 5, and cytokines.

Do you have to go to Mexico to get this stuff? No, we can give you a contact right here. It's actually someone you already know. Who? You, that's who. All these chemicals are types of nerve growth factors, chemicals you're already producing to keep your neurons sharp.

How to take advantage of the brain's own healing mechanism

For many years, brain researchers have understood that the creation and survival of brain cells may hinge on nerve growth factors. Growth factors, including neurotrophic brain proteins, are biochemical compounds that switch on the genes of stem cells so they develop into the right specific type of cell. They then help to guide those newly-generated cells to the appropriate part of the brain. Finally, they help maintain, protect, and repair brain cells once they're in place.

Ramon y Cajal, the pioneering brain researcher, who could not grow new brain cells, conjectured that the problem in adults may be an absence of the growth factors so abundant in the developing brain of a fetus. It turns out that adult brains do, indeed, produce growth factors and that these chemicals continue to play a role in brain cell maintenance and repair throughout life. Recent research has focused on identifying the different kinds of growth factor involved in maintaining different kinds of brain cells, and in learning how to manipulate or augment the brain's own growth factors to keep brain cells alive and healthy.

The brain's response to injuries is supplying crucial clues

The brain produces extra quantities — five to fifty times normal levels — of growth factors after a brain injury. Also, it has now been discovered that *glial* cells that help neurons to function properly also produce growth factors essential to the survival of neurons, and migrate to the site of a brain injury immediately after it occurs.

This evidence suggests the possibility that stroke or head-accident victims might recover more quickly by stimulating the brain's production of growth factors, or by somehow adding to what the brain is already doing to help itself. One line of current research is, in fact, exploring the feasibility of injecting growth factors into the site of a brain injury to help the brain recover more quickly. In animal experiments, even neurons apparently destroyed by having their axons cut (rendering them incapable of sending messages to other brain cells) are restored to full function if nerve growth factors are injected within three weeks after the damage.

How aged laboratory animals start to learn faster

Other experiments have shown that aged rats can regain youthful learning curves when growth factors are injected into the same frontal regions of the brain that degenerate in AD. Recently, researchers have also successfully grafted into rats cells that secrete growth factors on an ongoing basis, to prevent cognitive impairment before it even starts.

In the meantime, the news that you can really use is this: the "use it or lose it" principle applies to growth factors as well as to the regeneration of neurons. In fact, raised levels of growth factors may be the reason that an enriched environment enhances survival of newly generated brain cells, aids in recovery from stroke, and helps forestall dementias such as AD.

A person's own "go get 'em" attitude is the best brain medicine

It's been known for many years that an enriched environment — one providing extra physical, social, and mental stimulation — translates into improved performance on intelligence-type tests and into a bigger brain. In her pioneering studies, Marian Diamond attributed the larger brains of enriched-environment rats to larger neurons with richer-branching axons and dendrites and thicker myelin insulation. Later work found evidence for a larger number of neurons in an "enriched" brain as well, and evidence for a doubled rate of new brain-cell production under enriched conditions.

Why you should marry someone smarter than you are

Over the last ten years, a substantial body of research on humans has shown that a stimulating environment also has a strong effect on those all-important brain nutrients known as nerve growth factors. Proof began to accumulate starting with a 1990 study that revealed high levels of nerve growth factors in enriched-environment rats compared to standard-environment ones.

These findings are important for people worried about declines in learning ability and memory. The hippocampus, a brain structure central to those skills, is also one of the brain structures most strongly affected by AD. Physical exercise helps too. A subsequent study showed that rats with free access to a running wheel had increased levels of a neurotrophic-type growth factor than rats that had no chance to exercise. In this experiment, too, the extra growth factor molecules showed up in the hippocampus. Recent studies have proven that exercise increases growth factor levels in older men and women. So we now have proof that the findings about the relationship between an enriched environment and nerve growth factor levels in the brain apply to humans too.

Mood, mental maintenance, and sleep

Other recent findings have shed light on the connection between mood and cognitive maintenance, and on the connection between both those things and sleep. While you sleep, your body produces cell-regulating proteins called *cytokines*, part of your natural system for fighting diseases and maintaining brain cells. Cytokines also play a role in neurotransmitter systems important for mood and proper mental function, as well as for good sleep. So sleep deprivation can set a vicious spiral in motion, leading to further sleep problems and problems with mood, mental function, and general health. The moral is to take sleep problems seriously and to address their underlying cause.

Diet can affect brain growth

Other research has pointed to findings that a low-calorie diet helps you live longer, based on experiments with rodents. It also appears that it may help you stay smarter. Mice that are fed a restricted, low calorie diet have elevated levels of neural growth factors, and a higher rate of survival of newly-generated neurons. Also, a recently reported study of 1,423 participants in the Framingham Heart study revealed correlations between obesity and lower cognitive function in men, even after controlling for age, education, occupation, and health factors such as blood pressure.

REFERENCES FOR SECTION 3
Nerve growth factors and neurogenesis:
Altman, J., and G.D. Das. 1965. "Autoradiographic and histological evidence of postnatal hippocampal neurogenesis in rats." *Journal of Comparative Neurology* 124:319-36.

Bermon, S., et al. 1999. "Responses of total and free insulin-like growth factor-1 and insulin-like growth factor binding protein-3 after resistance exercise and training in elderly subjects." *Acta Physiologica Scandinavica* 165/1:51-6.

Bjorklund, A., and C. Svendsen. 1999. "Breaking the brain-blood barrier." *Nature* 397:569-70.

Bjornson, C.R., et al. 1999. "Turning brain into blood: a hematopoietic fate adopted by adult neural stem cells in vivo." *Science* 283:534-537.

Chadan, S.D., et al. 1999. "Influence of physical activity on plasma insulin-like growth factor-1and insulin-like growth factor binding proteins in healthy older women." *Mechanisms of Aging and Development* 109/1:21-34.

Dechant, G., and H. Neumann. 2002. "Neurotrophins." *Advances in Experimental Medical Biology* 513:303-34.

Edelman, G.M. 1987. *Neural Darwinism: The theory of neuronal group selection.* New York: Basic Books.

Eriksson P.S., et al. 1998. "Neurogenesis in the adult human hippocampus." *Nature Medicine* 4/11:1313-17.

Fischer, W., et al. 1991. "NGF improves spatial memory in aged rodents as a function of age." *Journal of Neuroscience* 11/7:1889-1906.

Gomez-Pinilla, F., V. So, and S.P Kesslak. 1998. "Spatial learning and physical activity contribute to the induction of fibroblast growth factor: neural substrates for increased cognition associated with exercise." *Neuroscience* 85/1:53-61.

Gould, E., et al. 1999. "Learning enhances adult neurogenesis in the hippocampal formation." *Nature Neuroscience* 2/3:260-5.

Heerssen, H.M., and R.A. Segal. 2002. "Location, location, location: a spatial view of neurotrophin signal transduction." *Trends in Neuroscience* 253:160-5.

Johansson, C.B., et al. 1999. "Neural stem cells in the adult human brain." *Experimental Cell Research* 253/2:733-6.

Kuhn, H.G., T.D. Palmer, and E. Fuchs. 2001. "Adult neurogenesis: a compensatory mechanism for neuronal damage." *European Archives of Psychiatry and Clinical Neuroscience* 251/4:152-8.

Lacroix. S., and M.H. Tuszynski. 2000. "Neurotrophic factors and gene therapy in spinal cord injury." *Neurorehabilitation and Neural Repair* 14/4:265-75.

Martinez-Serrano, A., and A. Bjorklund. 1998. "Ex vivo nerve growth factor gene transfer to the basal forebrain in presymptomatic middle-aged rats prevents the development of cholinergic neuron atrophy during aging." *Proceedings of the National Academy of Science USA* 95:1858-63.

Morrison, J.H., and P.R. Hof. 2002. "Selective vulnerability of corticocortical and hippocampal circuits in aging and Alzheimer's disease." *Progress in Brain Research* 136:467-86.

Neeper, S.A., et al. 1995. "Exercise and brain neurotrophins." *Nature* 375:109.

Rosenblad, C., D.K. Kirik, and A. Bjorklund. 2000. "Sequential administration of GDNF into the substantia nigra and striatum." *Experimental Neurology* 61/2:503-16.

Russo-Neustadt, A. 2003. "Brain-derived neurotrophic factor, behavior, and new directions for the treatment of mental disorders." *Seminars in Clinical Neuropsychiatry* 8/2:109-18.

Scharff, C., et al. 2000. "Targeted neuronal death affects neuronal replacement and vocal behavior in adult songbirds." *Neuron* 25:481-92.

Sinson, G., M. Voddi, and T.K. McIntosh. 1995. "Nerve growth factor administration attenuates cognitive but not neurobehavioral motor dysfunction or hippocampal cell loss following fluid-percussion brain injury in rats." *Journal of Neurochemistry* 65/5:2209-16.

Environmental enrichment and brain plasticity:
Bennett, E.L., et al. 1974. "Effects of successive environments on brain measures." *Physiology and Behavior* 12/4:621-31.

Bonaiuto, S., E. Rocca, and A. Lippi. 1990. "Impact of education and occupation on the prevalence of Alzheimer's disease (AD) and multi-infarct dementia in Macerata Province, Italy." *Neurology* 40 (Suppl. 1):346.

Clayton, N.S., and J.R. Krebs. 1994. "Hippocampal growth and attrition in birds affected by experience." *Proceedings of the National Academy of Science USA* 91:7410-14.

Connor, J.R., and M.C. Diamond. 1982. "A comparison of dendritic spine number and type on pyramidal neurons of the visual cortex of old rats from social or isolated environments." *The Journal of Comparative Neurology* 210:99-106.

Cotman, C.W., and N.C. Berchtold. 2002. "Exercise: a behavioral intervention to enhance brain health and plasticity." *Trends in Neuroscience* 25/6:295-301

Dartigues, J.F., et al. 1992. "Occupation during life and memory performance in nondemented French elderly community residents." *Neurology* 42:1697-1701.

van Dellen, A., et al. 2000. "Delaying the onset of Huntington's in mice." *Nature* 404:721-2.

Diamond, M., and J. Hopson. 1998. *Magic Trees of the Mind: How to nurture your child's intelligence, creativity, and healthy emotions from birth through adolescence.* New York: Plume.

Elias, M.F., et al. 2003. "Lower cognitive function in the presence of obesity and hypertension: the Framingham heart study." *International Journal of Obesity and Related Metabolic Disorders* 27/2:260-8.

Freidland, R.P. 1993. "Epidemiology, education, and the ecology of Alzheimer's disease." *Neurology* 43:246-9.

Friedland, R.P., et al. 2001. "Patients with Alzheimer's disease have reduced activities in midlife compared with healthy control-group members." *Proceedings of the National Academy of Sciences* 98/6:3440-5.

Gatz, M., et al. 1994. "Dementia: not just a search for the gene." *The Gerontologist* 34/2:251-5.

Gould, E., et al. 1999. "Learning enhances adult neurogenesis in the hippocampal formation." *Nature Neuroscience* 2/3:260-5.

Held, R. 1965. "Plasticity in sensory motor systems." *Scientific American* 213:84-94.

Jacobs, B., M. Schall, and A.B. Scheibel. 1993. "A quantitative dendritic analysis of Wernicke's area in humans." *The Journal of Comparative Neurology* 327:97-111.

Kelche, C., et al. 1995. "The effects of intrahippocampal grafts, training, and postoperative housing on behavioral recovery after septohippocampal damage in the rat." *Neurobiology of Learning and Memory* 63/2:155-66.

Korczyn, A.D, E. Kahana, and Y. Galper. 1991. "Epidemiology of dementia in Ashkelon, Israel." *Neuroepidemiology* 10:100.

Lee, J., K.B. Seroogy, and M.P. Mattson. 2002. "Dietary restriction enhances neurotrophin expression and neurogenesis in the hippocampus of adult mice." *Journal of Neurochemistry* 80/3:539-47.

Lendvai, B., et al. 2000. "Experience-dependent plasticity of dendritic spines in the developing rat barrel cortex in vivo." *Nature* 404:876-81.

Marshall, L., and J. Born. 2002. "Brain-immune interactions in sleep." *International Review of Neurobiology* 52:93-131.

von Melchner, L., S.L. Pallas, and M. Sur. 2000. "Visual behavior mediated by retinal projections directed to the auditory pathway." *Nature* 404:871-5.

Mohammed, A.K., et al. 1990. "Environmental influence on behavior and nerve growth factor in the brain." *Brain Research* 528/1:62-70.

Mortimer, J.A., and A.B. Graves. 1993. "Education and other socioeconomic determinants of dementia and Alzheimer's disease." *Neurology* 43 (Suppl. 4):S39-44.

Pham, T.M., et al. 1999. "Effects of environmental enrichment on cognitive function and hippocampal NGF in the brains of non-handled rats." *Behavioural Brain Research* 103/1:63-70.

van Praag, H., G. Kempermann, and F.H. Gage. 1999. "Running increases cell proliferation and neurogenesis in the adult mouse dentate gyrus." *Nature Neuroscience* 2/3:266-70.

Raiha, I., et al. 1998. "Environmental differences in twin pairs discordant for Alzheimer's disease." *Journal of Neurology, Neurosurgery, and Psychiatry* 65/5:785-7.

Rosenzweig, M.R., and E.L. Bennett. 1996. "Psychobiology of plasticity: effects of training and experience on brain and behavior." *Behavioural Brain Research* 78:57-65.

Schofield, P.W., et al. 1995. "The age at onset of Alzheimer's disease and an intracranial area measurement: a relationship." *Archives of Neurology* 52:95-8.

Schaie, KW. 1994. "The course of adult intellectual development." *American Psychologist* 49:304-13.

Sharma, J., A. Angelucci, and M. Sur. 2000. "Induction of visual orientation modules in auditory cortex." *Nature* 404:841-7.

Snowdon, D.A., et al. 1989. "Years of life with good and poor mental function in the elderly." *Journal of Clinical Epidemiology* 42:1055-66.

Snowdon, D.A., et al. 1996. "Linguistic ability in early life and cognitive function and Alzheimer's disease in late life." *JAMA* 275/7:528-32.

Stein, D.G., S. Brailowsky, and B. Will. 1997. *Brain Repair*. Oxford: Oxford University Press.

Stern, Y., et al. 1992. "Inverse relationship between education and parietotemporal perfusion deficit in Alzheimer's disease." *Annals of Neurology* 32/3:371-5.

Stern, Y., et al. 1994. "Influence of education and occupation on the incidence of Alzheimer's disease." *JAMA* 271/13:1004-10.

Swaab, D.F. 1991. "Brain aging and Alzheimer's disease, 'wear and tear' versus 'use it or lose it.'" *Neurobiology of Aging* 12:317-24.

Swaab, D.F. 1998. "Reduced neuronal activity and reactivation in Alzheimer's disease." *Progress in Brain Research* 117:343-77.

Verghese, J., et al. 2003. "Leisure activities and the risk of dementia in the elderly." *The New England Journal of Medicine* 348/25:2508-16.

Wilson, R.S., et al. 2002. "Cognitive activity and incident AD in a population-based sample of older persons." *Neurology* 59:1910-14.

Wilson, R.S., et al. 2002. "Participation in cognitively stimulating activities and risk of incident Alzheimer's disease." *JAMA* 287/6:742-8.

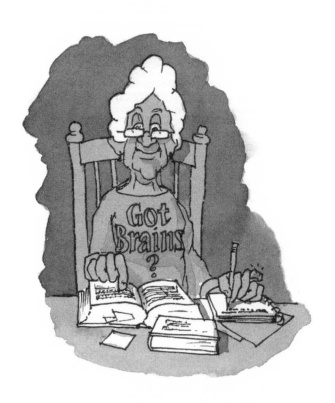

SECTION 4

MENTAL CONDITIONING EXERCISES

The brain exercises that follow are targeted to stimulate crucial functions and pathways that relate directly to professional performance and personal quality of life. The six behavioral categories, listed on the prior page, recruit a wide variety of the brain's circuits and the many pathways that connect them. The exercises within each category are designed to stimulate those specific clusters of practical cognitive skills used every day.

In reality the brain needs combinations of its tools to respond to the world. Therefore, for best results, we suggest that you tackle the types of exercise that you think may be hard for you. Every brain is as different as every face so some types of mental exercises will come easier than others to everyone.

In that sense, the weight-lifter's mantra "no pain, no gain" applies to mental exercise also. But the good news is that your brain loves its job. It will build just as much muscle while you are having a good time playing with these mental puzzlers as it would memorizing a list of prime numbers. So enjoy yourself. Nobody's watching.

Within each exercise we have inserted two hints, called "helping hands" (they are marked by this symbol ☞). Refer to them to ease your way to exploring a skill you may have shied away from because you thought you were not "good at it."

You will find these two optional helping hands printed upside down in smaller type. Our goal is to help you break up any cases of mental block that might have set in as you confront each new task so you can enjoy being successful. The brain rewards completion of a sustained mental challenge by releasing a natural substance called *serotonin*, which imparts a sense of emotional well-being. In effect, the brain rewards efforts to sharpen its own skills. Since we wouldn't want you to miss out on either benefit the helping hands will keep you going without having to look at the answer. They are also marked with an image of a hand so you can avoid reading them unless and until you find yourself completely stuck. See page 193 for solutions.

The first of these suggestions for getting started toward a solution is printed upside down following the instructions for that exercise.

The second suggestion is printed upside down at the bottom of that page.

Visual & Mechanical

RUBE MONKEYBERG

Rube is cranking the wheel in a clockwise direction, causing the elaborate collection of connected wheels and pulleys to rotate the four cogged wheels at the end. These, in turn, will cause the four toothed plates, numbered 1, 2, 3, 4, to move. Only two of them will move toward each other and touch. Which two are they? Par is $2^{1}/_{2}$ minutes.

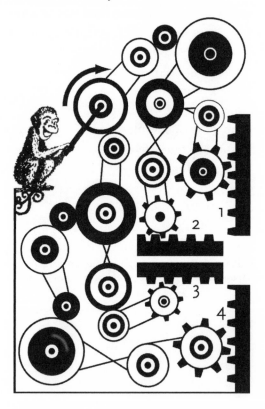

Pulley belts rotate both wheels in the same direction, except when belts are crossed.

When you get to the cogged wheels their rotation will slide the cogged rail one way or the other. For example, rail number one slides up.

CUBE CUTUP

Imagine that this block measures 3" x 3" x 3" and that it has designs on all six sides. Can you answer these questions?

a. How many cuts are needed to convert the block into 1" cubes?

b. How many 1" cubes will you have?

c. How many 1" cubes have a design on: 4 sides? 3 sides? 2 sides? 1 side?

d. How many cubes have no design on them?

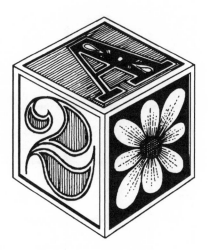

 c is an even number.

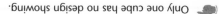 Only one cube has no design showing.

137

WINDOW BOXES

Lady Aster tired of the plant arrangement in the window of her country home. She insisted that the gardener change it so that two plants would always be situated in each horizontal, vertical, and the two corner-to-corner diagonal rows. To her astonishment it took him only two minutes and he only moved five plants! Can you best the gardener's time?

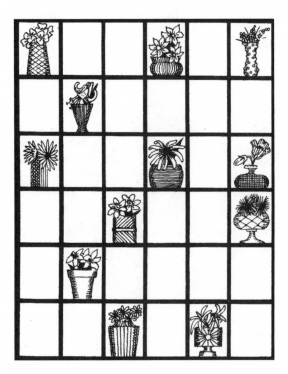

☞ Move the center plant on the third row from the top straight down to the bottom row.

☞ The bottom row is completed when the plant on the right is moved one row straight up.

BLOCK PARTY

Five of these six blocks are exactly the same. Study them and try to figure out the answers to the following questions:

1. On one of the three cubes to the left, the numbers on opposite sides have been switched. Is it A, B, or C?

2. Which two numbers were switched?

3. What number on cube E is against cube D?

4. What number is against cube F?

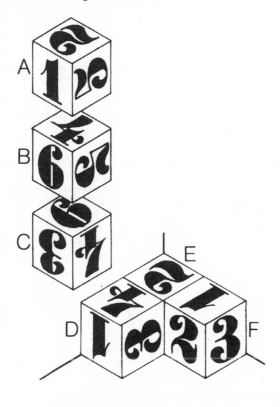

☞ Figure out what number is opposite the number 2.

☞ In B, the base of the 4 sits on the top of the 6, but not in C. Why?

139

MATCH PATCH

1. Make three equal squares using these four whole matches and the four half matches.

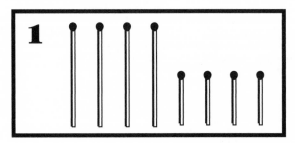

 Think of a bird's eye view of three adjoining baseball diamonds.

2. Remove three matches and end up with three triangle

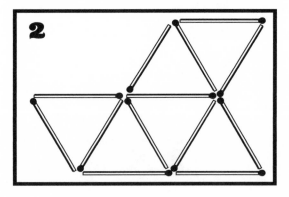

 Think "outside the box" by thinking big.

 #2 First, create the Great Pyramid.

 #1 Start with two big Xs.

STACK ROOM

This puzzle is harder to do if you don't touch it or write on it. See if you can figure out:

A. How many stacks of white tiles are needed to fill the center area, and how many white stacks are needed to fill in around the outside edges of the room?

B. How many black stacks for the center area, and for the edge?

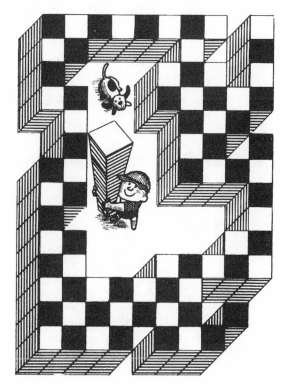

☞ Use arithmetic. Count the number of stacks on each full side. Divide by two for white or black tiles. If you need the next step, see the next hint.

☞ Now count the number of stacks that show in each row and subtract them from the number of stacks in a full row.

LOGIC & MEMORY

PARTY HATS

Two men, Allen and Wally, and a woman, Carolyn, have volunteered to play a "logic" game at a party. They are blindfolded and a party hat is put on each of their heads. The three are told that when the blindfolds are removed, each is to raise a hand if she or he sees a striped hat on one or more heads, and to lower the hand when he or she logically figures out whether he or she is wearing a striped hat. Unknown to the players, they're all wearing striped hats. When the blindfolds are removed, all hands go up

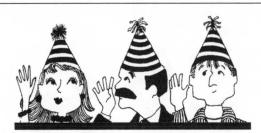

Shortly afterward, Carolyn lowers her hand.

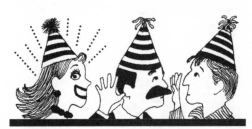

How did she know she was wearing a striped hat?

 Carolyn waited a few moments to see if Allen and Wally were seeing more than one striped hat.

 What would Allen and Wally have done if Carolyn's hat was unstriped?

MIND'S EYE

Read these instructions first before starting. Study every detail in the boxes (below, left) for about a minute. When you think you've implanted the pictures in your mind's eye, cover the ten boxes on the left side and draw the objects in the correct boxes at the right on on a separate sheet of paper. Eight is excellent; six good; five fair.

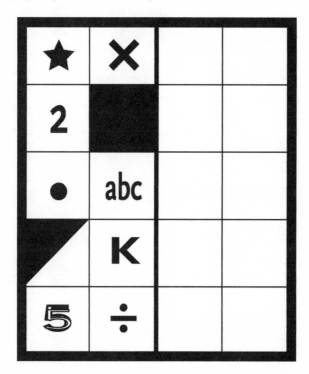

 It is OK to peek, cover it, and try again.

 Note how many "peeks" you needed to get them all. Let someone else try.

HAIRY PROBLEM

Don't tear your hair out over this one! Bob and Harry have different color hair. Tom's hair is the same color as Dick's and Tom is on the right side of Bob and on the left side of Harry, whose hair is the same color as Tony's. Which boy is which?

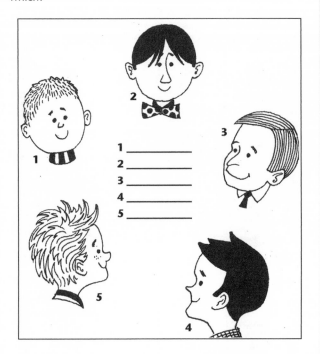

1 _____
2 _____
3 _____
4 _____
5 _____

 Tony and Dick are wearing ties.

 Bob has a crew cut.

HOUSE GUEST

In each of these four houses (A, B, C, and D) lives a student. Each student has a favorite academic subject. Three of them have pets, and one has Sir Rodney as a houseguest. Study the following information and see if you can answer the two questions at the end.

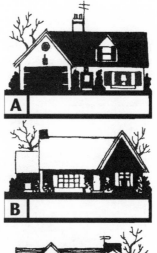

1. The student in house C studies physics.

2. The dog lives next door to the horse.

3. John is great at math.

4. Ed lives between the horse owner and the physics student.

5. Tina lives next door to the cat owner.

6. The student in house D studies philosophy.

7. Lulu's cat fights with her English-student neighbor's dog.

8. Sir Rodney cannot stand pets.

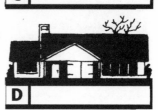

In which house does John live?

In which house is Sir Rodney visiting?

When you think you have figured out where the pets live, you may want to write the pet into the box below each house with a pet, and "Sir Rodney" in the remaining house.

 Where does the guy who likes math live?

 Doesn't it seem likely that a British aristocrat would be the guest of a philosopher?

145

DRESS-UP TIME

Three little girls, Allyson, Daryl, and Karen are spending a rainy day playing dress-up. They have each brought together some of their mothers' "attic" clothes for the occasion. Each girl is wearing a dress and a hat brought by two of the other girls. The one who is wearing Karen's hat is wearing Daryl's dress. Who is wearing Allyson's dress?

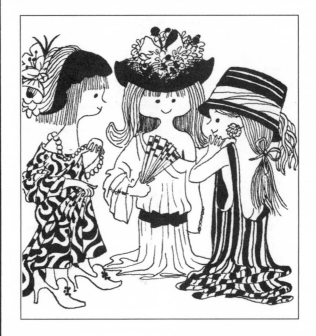

 Allyson is wearing Karen's hat.

 Daryl is wearing Karen's dress.

FLOWER SHOW

The annual Summer Flower Show was held in the small town of South Yarmouth. Four members of the garden club, Angie, Bobbi, Karen, and Lorraine, displayed arrangements of their favorite flowers. One focused on white carnations, two selected roses, and one showed her special pansies. Mrs. Fellows, Mrs. Dickinson, Mrs. Kennedy, and Miss Pappas were very pleased when they learned they had each won an award. From the following clues, you should be able to tell each woman's full name and the type of flower each exhibited.

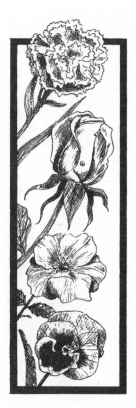

1. Lorraine's exhibit was next to the woman who displayed the white carnations.

2. Karen and Miss Pappas exhibited different flowers.

3. Mrs. Fellows and Mrs. Dickinson displayed different flowers.

4. Bobbi and Mrs. Dickinson had displays that showed flowers in many different colors.

5. Angie's exhibit was three tables away from Lorraine's and across the aisle from the woman who displayed pansies.

6. Mrs. Fellows and Karen are related.

7. Angie and Mrs. Dickinson are close friends.

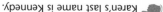 Karen's last name is Kennedy.

CARD SENSE

1. Four cards are dealt. There is an ace under an ace. Over a diamond there is a club. A queen is over an ace, and under a heart there is a diamond. Also, a diamond is over a heart, and a queen is under an ace. What are the four cards?

2. Three cards lie face down. A heart is to the left of a diamond. A four is to the right of a king. A seven is to the left of a spade, and a spade is to the left of a diamond. What are the three cards?

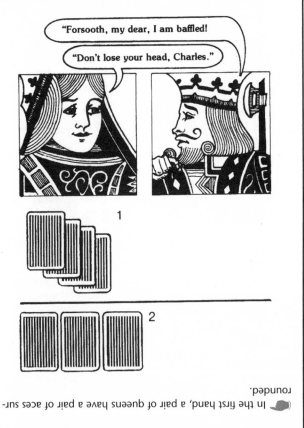

"Forsooth, my dear, I am baffled!

"Don't lose your head, Charles."

1

2

☞ In the first hand, a pair of queens have a pair of aces surrounded.

☞ In the second hand, the highest card is in the middle.

DIVERGENT THINKING

VIN ORDINAIRE

Group A shows three empty glasses and three full glasses of wine. What is the smallest number of glasses you must pick up to create the arrangement shown in group B?

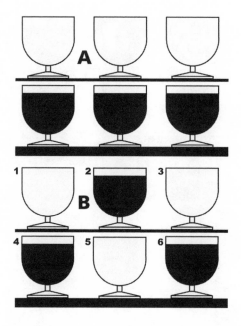

☞ The 5th glass asks "what is another word for 'decant'?"

☞ Glass #5 says, "What's the simplest way for me to lose weight?"

PARTICULAR PAIRS

The twenty pictures below may be placed into ten pairs that are logically associated. Some might be paired with more than one picture—the mouse, cat, dog, bird, and pig are all animals, for example. However, when logically paired there should be no leftovers that are not related.

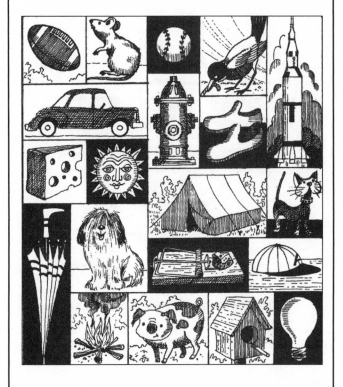

 A weird pairing would match cheese and pig because they're both food.

 A logical pairing would match campfire and tent.

POSSIBLE PAIRS

Make six pairs out of these twelve different items. Use each picture once and don't leave out any pictures. Pair them so that all seven are the best combinations, based on whatever similarities make most sense to you. There is no "correct" solution; some possibilities are given on the answer page.

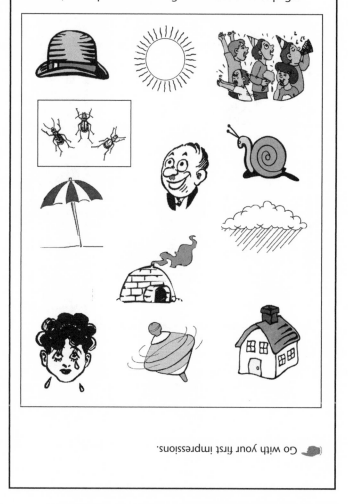

☞ Go with your first impressions.

☞ Try turning the page upside down and pair them again. That will engage your literal right brain to look for shapes.

151

PATTERN & PATHFINDING

TANGLE TRACE

The five objects shown in the small boxes are associated with the five pictures in the large box. Draw a continuous line from each small box to the picture it best matches. You may not cross a line you've already drawn.

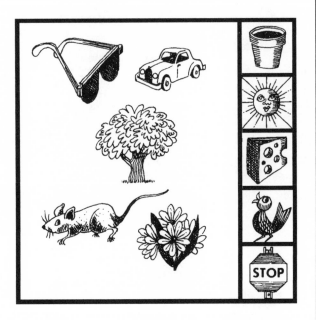

 The bird has the shortest trip.

 The flowerpot has an outside chance of finding its partner.

NUMBER SEARCH

Hidden in this mass of numbers is one special combination for you to find. Look for a six to the right, a four above, a two below, and a nine to the left of a particular number. What is the number?

9	0	6	3	7	4	0	4	3	5	7	6
5	2	4	0	9	5	2	7	9	2	0	4
7	8	1	6	2	6	3	6	4	8	9	5
6	5	2	8	9	5	6	5	9	6	3	1
7	9	0	4	3	7	1	8	2	7	5	0
3	4	6	1	8	6	3	5	0	1	2	3
1	8	7	2	4	5	2	7	8	9	1	6
0	3	1	6	5	9	1	0	2	3	4	5
7	6	9	8	2	3	8	5	9	6	7	3
1	4	6	3	0	9	2	0	4	3	1	9
5	6	2	1	4	6	1	9	7	6	4	2
3	0	7	5	3	0	4	8	2	5	1	7
7	2	4	2	1	9	5	6	3	9	5	6
1	8	3	6	5	8	3	1	2	8	4	0
4	6	2	7	0	7	6	9	4	6	1	9
3	8	0	9	1	5	6	2	3	5	2	7

 Try scanning for only one of the numbers.

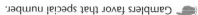 Gamblers favor that special number.

FLOWER DISARRANGEMENT

One picture and one silhouette exactly match the picture in box 1. Careful! Some of the differences are quite small.

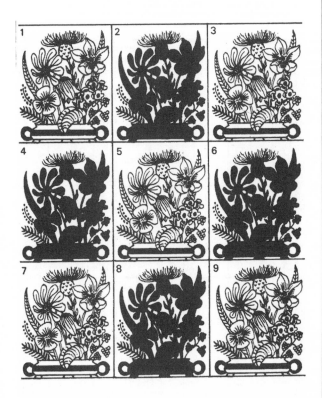

 Look closely at the left side of the flower arrangement in picture 9.

 Look closely at the right side of the flower arrangement in silhouette 8.

MATCH BOXES

The designs in the seven boxes to the right of the picture match seven squares in the picture. Each square in the grid that is laid over the picture can be coded by a letter (across the top) and a number (down the side). Match each box with the identical square in the picture. As you make a match, write the "locater code" beneath the box. In case you wondered, all the boxes are right side up.

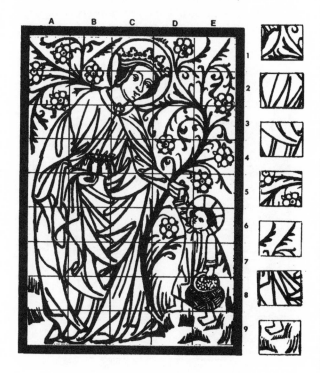

☞ Did you write "E-9" below the box at the bottom?

☞ Does the square in the upper right-hand corner of the picture match any of the boxes?

MISSING PIECES

This old woodcut was reproduced onto ceramic tiles, which were bought by a large museum to exhibit as a fine example of Dutch art. Eight tiles were stolen by marauding Tzlopkitlians, but they were recovered in time for the opening of the exhibit. Can you help the aggravated museum curator figure out where the four loose tiles at the top and the four at the bottom should be placed to complete the picture? He's particularly annoyed because he has to rotate each tile to make a match. Write your answers in the small boxes attached to each lost piece using the grid locations (A-1, for example).

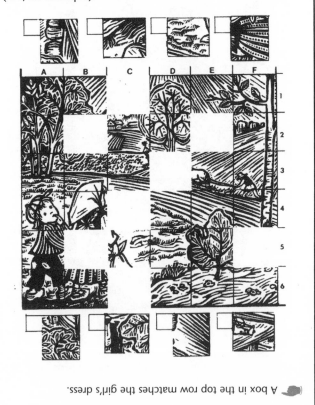

☞ A box in the top row matches the girl's dress.

☞ The tile with the missing tree trunk is upside down in the bottom row.

MENTAL JIGSAW

This is a reproduction of a Nootka Eskimo woodcarving showing a lightning-snake, a wolf, and a killer whale. Write the number of each piece that has been cut out of the picture in the circle where it should go. In this exercise you may not get them all because the design is abstract and the pieces are rotated. Nine correct answers is an excellent score. Seven is good. Five is fair.

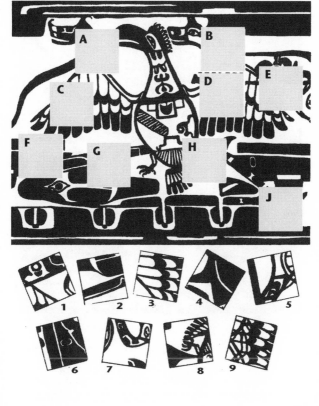

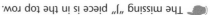

☞ A piece with part of the lightning-snake is in the bottom row.

☞ The missing "J" piece is in the top row.

PLAY THE SYMBOLS

Eight symbols are arranged in this grid seemingly at random. You must study all the variations to figure out which symbol should be placed in the box containing the question mark.

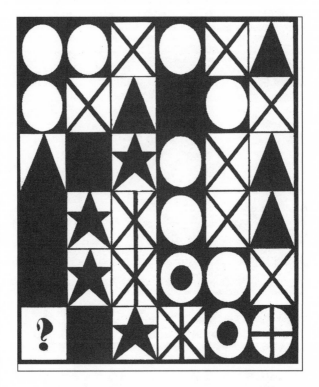

 Begin at the top working left to right.

 Assign number values to the symbols. The "X" symbol is a "2."

TANGRAM

If you cut the square (below left) along the lines drawn
through it, you would have seven geometric shapes.
Figures like those below can be made by arranging the
seven pieces in different ways, using each piece only once.
However, four of the pieces used in Figures A through E
could not possibly have been cut from this particular
square. When you find these four, put their numbers in the
boxes below.

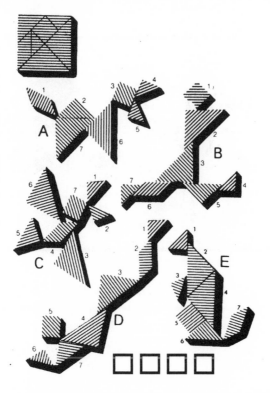

☞ Pay attention to the direction of the lines on the pieces in
the figures and the lines on the corresponding pieces in the
square.

☞ Check piece 6 in figure B. Are the lines running in correct
direction?

LANGUAGE

PHUNNEY PHONETICS

On a trip to the seashore, our otherwise erudite British guest was utterly baffled by this sign. It's composed of two common English words. When used in various combinations in other common words, these letters, singly or in combination, sound completely different. Can you help our friend find out whether or not this happens to be on his shopping list.

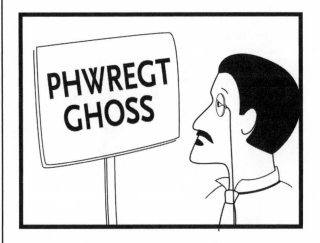

 Think of all the ways to write an "F" sound.

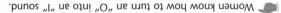 Women know how to turn an "O" into an "I" sound.

Word Mix-up

When the eighteen pairs of letters around this grid are correctly assembled within the grid, two four-letter, two five-letter, two six-letter and two seven-letter words will be constructed. Each corner letter is part of two words, crossword fashion. You may use each pair of letters only once.

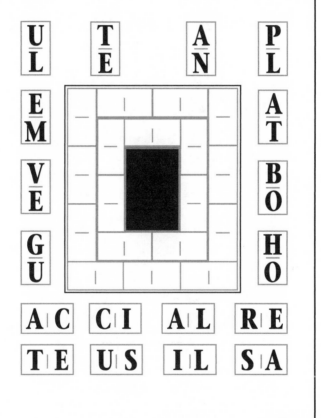

☞ The "PL" letter pair fits into the upper left-hand corner of the grid.

☞ One of the four-letter words is BUSH.

161

LETTER LOGIC

There is a logical reason why the words in this list are placed in the order shown. Only one of the four words below the dotted line will complete the list. Can you select the right one and write it on the dotted line?

NEGOTIATION
REBATED
TRANSLATE
ARCHDUCHESS
STRUGGLING
TRESPASSERS
PROMOTE
CONDUCTOR

– – – – – – – – –

FOLLOW   EVINCE
DADDY   ROTATE

 The first word on the list would not have been chosen if there had been more of them.

 "Oh, oh!" exclaimed the detective when he read the last two words on the list.

TWISTS & TURNS

Arguments begin when one word leads to another, and in this puzzle words not only lead to each other, but often overlap. If you start in slot #1 with the right word and continue clockwise you should have little trouble completing the circle with nine additional words. Each word starts in a numbered slot that corresponds to the number of the clue.

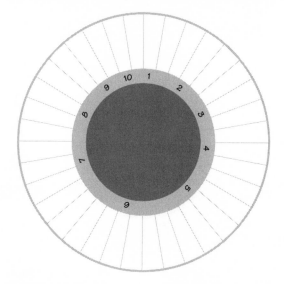

1. Cheese gadget sounds larger
2. Altered steer succinctly
3. Whimsically erects a mystery
4. Pensioner withdrew from the fray
5. Misleading sardine (two words)
6. Highly skilled circus employee
7. The senator was transformed without a cooking fuel
8. Innovative Ron follows neither
9. Caring differently about Belmont business?
10. Thankless person tearing apart the place!

 #5 is a Commie!

 #7 is often found in camping kits.

Brrrrr!

Arguments begin when one word leads to another, and in this puzzle words not only lead to each other, but often overlap. If you start in slot #1 with the right word and continue clockwise you should have little trouble completing the circle with eleven additional words. Each word starts in a numbered slot that corresponds to the number of the clue.

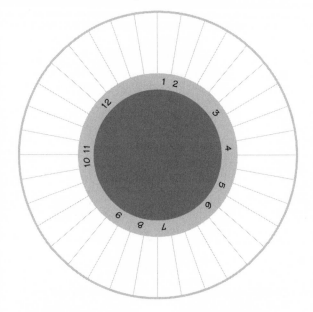

1. Shakespearian season of discontent
2. Bank charge
3. Not active
4. Prickling sensation often associated with backbones
5. Astronaut and senator
6. Group of nine

7. Hold in esteem
8. Stuck in the mud
9. Warning signal (two words)
10. Small-sized type
11. Heavenly openers
12. Specter; a mere semblance

 You can also use a #10 to shoot marbles.

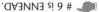 # 6 is ENNEAD.

LADDERGRAM/CHANGEUPS

Start at the top word and change one letter in each word as you go down the ladder. We have already put in a couple of words under "skirt" to get you started. Letters do not change position in any word. The bottom words, when solved and unscrambled, will form a well-known saying. The word "is" in the top box is used in the saying but not in the ladder.

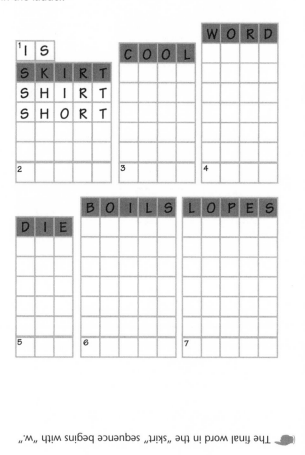

☞ The final word in the "skirt" sequence begins with "w."

☞ The final word in the "lopes" sequence begins with "m" and ends with "y."

165

WORD SPIRAL

The names of the foods listed opposite fit into the spiral grid. Beginning at the star, spell a food with its first letter in a circle and its last letter in the next circle. Thus, the last letter of a word will be the first letter of the following word. You will always be writing from left to right. When you reach a corner, turn the puzzle one fourth of a turn counterclockwise to continue. Continue inserting words in a spiral fashion until you reach the center box and all of the words have been put in the grid. We've given you a head start to send you on your way.

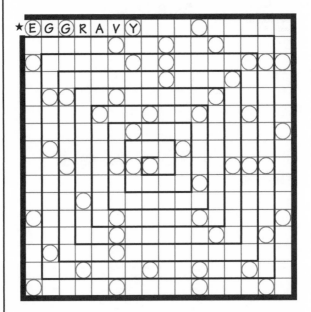

 Find where "tenderloin" and "Worcestershire" fit, and add them to the grid.

Word Spiral Word List

3	kabob	oatmeal
egg	liver	risotto
ham	roast	tapioca
	salad	
4	taffy	8
edam	toast	dressing
lamb	tripe	noodles
meat	wafer	sandwich
nuts	yeast	tortilla
peas		turnover
pork	6	
roll	cheese	9
slaw	éclair	appetizer
soup	muffin	doughnuts
stew	olives	entremets
tart	omelet	Roquefort
yolk	ragout	
	tomato	10
5	turkey	tenderloin
aspic	yogurt	
bread		14
dough	7	Worcestershire
gravy	biscuit	
gumbo	ketchup	

 Working backward, the innermost word in the spiral is "olives."

167

WORDS ANY-WAY

The letter grid below contains the names of at least twenty-nine countries. To spell a country, you must choose letters moving from one box to an adjacent box, but the move may be vertical, horizontal, or diagonal, up or down. You may change direction, or not, as you move from one letter to the next. Every letter in the grid is used at least once, and some are used more than once, but never twice in a row. As you find the names of countries write them in the spaces below. The number spaces indicate the number of letters in each name. Place the grid location of the first letter in the grid box. We've given you a super hint as to how to play this game. A2-A1-B1-C2-B3-C3-D3 spells BELGIUM.

	A	B	C	D	E	F	G	H	
	E	L	N	E	L	O	E	C	1
	B	Y	G	A	R	M	L	Y	2
	A	I	U	M	T	A	P	R	3
	N	E	B	R	I	N	U	E	4
	O	R	O	Y	T	S	C	B	5
	S	W	A	S	B	E	U	A	6
	I	O	L	I	R	G	L	N	7
	M	N	D	E	A	Z	I	A	8

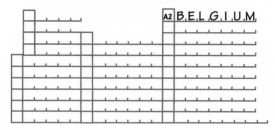

A2 B.E.L.G.I.U.M.

☞ The first letter of a four-letter country begins with C5.

☞ The first letter of a nine-letter country begins with C2 and uses one letter four times!

COMPUTATION

ANTIQUE ACCOUNTING

The Gotrock's attended a "collectibles" antique show and got carried away with their purchases. The items for sale were exhibited in groups of various price categories. One from each group is shown here. Of the eight price categories, Frau Gotrock bought five items from one group, four from another, and three from another. Herr Gotrock bought two from another, and one from a fifth group. They spent a total of $260. Can you figure out which price groups they chose items from, and how many items they bought in each group?

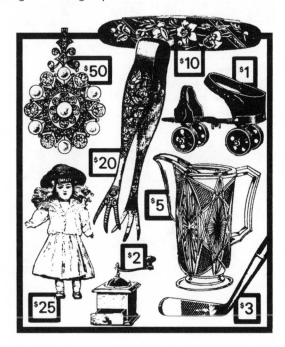

 They bought nothing from the $10 price group.

 The five items from one group cost $25 more than the two items from another group.

SYMBOLATICS

Each symbol represents a number between one and nine. Identical symbols represent the same number. When two symbols are together they represent a two-figure number. Each dot between symbols represents either a plus, minus, multiplication, or division sign. Each equation has the same answer, as shown in the column at the right. Can you match the symbols with their correct numbers?

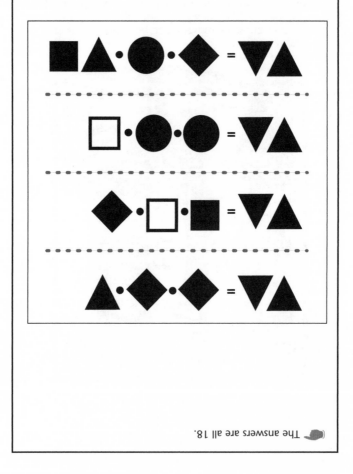

 The answers are all 18.

 Try using the ÷ and the + in the top row. No more .÷'s after that.

MISSING DIGITS

There is a definite reason why the numbers have been placed in the grids in the positions shown. Puzzle A follows a certain formula for obtaining the last number in each horizontal row. Puzzle B has its own special formula. Can you correctly fill in each final box?

A

12	4	64
9	6	9
17	11	?

What do the numbers in the top row have in common with the numbers in the middle row, and thus with the numbers in the bottom row?

B

A	B	C	D	E	F	G
2	4	12	8	40	12	?

Look at the boxes in the following sequence: ABC, CDE, EFG.

 B. Add first, then multiply.

 A. In each row, subtract the second number from the first to start finding the third number.

MATCH STICKLERS

These exercises are designed to recruit both hemispheres of the brain simultaneously. The left brain's temporal lobe will process the arithmetic. (If you know enough arithmetic to notice that all these equations are incorrect, you know enough to solve them.) The right hemisphere will visualize how moving only one of the matchsticks can convert one number, or math sign, into another.

As you see, for example: The number 1 is made of two matches end to end; The 4 has 4 matches (but swing one down and, presto! you make an 11); Remove one of the the 7 matches in the 8 and you make a 6; The 0 requires 6 matches, but add one in the middle and it is an 8; Move one of the 5 matches in the 5 and you have made a 3.

The same principle applies to the mathematical signs. They are made of one or two matches. The / stands for division (cross it with another match and you make a multiplication sign). Add one to the minus sign to make a plus sign. Use your visual imagination. HINT: In all the examples of Match Sticklers shown here the = sign remains intact.

Like all puzzles that use multiple cognitive processes, there can be more than one solution to some of these. Once you get into them they become as hard to resist as a bowl of peanuts. If you need help getting started please don't hesitate to check out the numbered hint printed upside down on this and the following page instead of turning to Solutions page 189.

Your task, in each of these seven exercises, is to move one, and only one, match to make the numbers on both sides of the equals sign form a balanced equation.

Ladies and gentlemen, start your visual-math engines!

1.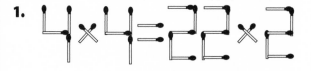

Remember what the instructions, above, said about the 4?

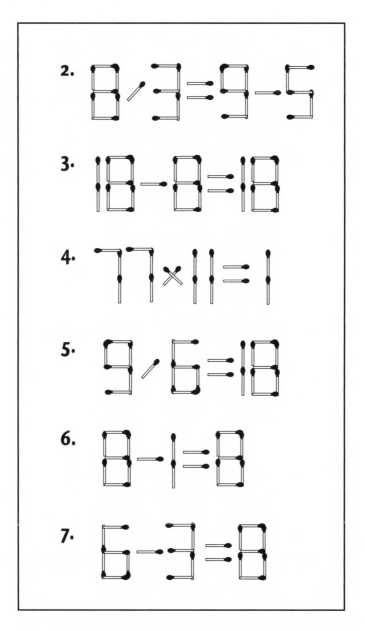

APPENDIX

If You Do Have Alzheimer's Disease

Current and future medications for combatting AD

One of the earliest theories about the cause of AD is that the disease stems from problems with the brain system that produces and responds to the chemical *acetylcholine,* a vital "memory" neurotransmitter. This theory is based partly on the fact that the cognitive skills of attention and memory that acetylcholine supports are some of the first skills that deteriorate in AD. More decisively, biopsies of the brains of AD patients show that it is mainly the neurons of the *cholinergic* system (the network of brain cells producing and responding to acetylcholine) that are harmed or destroyed early in the disease's progression. Also, levels of acetylcholine are lowest in AD patients with the most severe cognitive problems.

The notion that AD could be caused by a shortage of acetylcholine has led to the development of drugs that raise its levels within the brain. They do this by blocking the enzyme that breaks down acetylcholine after it has been released into the synapse (the communication junction between brain cells). This should, in theory, raise acetylcholine levels and help ensure the survival of neurons in the cholinergic system.

Drugs that inhibit the enzyme that breaks down acetylcholine have already been developed and are available by prescription. Donepezil, marketed under the brand name *Aricept*, is already available by prescription though it does not effectively slow down the course of developing dementia. Some other drugs, including rivastigmine (brand name *Exelon*) and metrifonate are undergoing or have undergone trials and are becoming available in the United States. Like antidepressants, some of these drugs also raise levels of the serotonin neurotransmitter, which tends to improve mood.

There is no clear scientific evidence that drugs that work on the cholinergic system are to be effective in slowing the progression of AD, and they are certainly not cures. As placebo or not, their clinical effect is said to work in the early stages before the symptoms become too severe. If so, early detection would help to maximize their effectiveness.

What the genetic research tells us

Along with increasingly sophisticated brain-imaging technology, the mapping of the human genome has fueled an explosion of knowledge about the brain. The more accurately geneticists can identify exactly which genes do what, the better neuroscientists can tease out the causes of physical and mental illnesses such as Parkinson's, depression, AD, and so on — on a genetic level.

In the case of AD, several genetic risk factors have been identified. Humans have about 80,000 genes, which contain the recipes used to manufacture all the many types of proteins that build and maintain our bodies. The genes are contained in structures called chromosomes. A full set of chromosomes is present in each cell in the body. A defective gene on chromosome 21, which builds a protein known as APP, has been argued to cause some forms of AD. People with this mutant gene are very likely to develop the amyloid deposits characteristic of brains that show AD-type degeneration.

Another gene found to be involved in AD is called (appropriately enough) *presenilin*. A mutated form of this gene also results in increased production of the substance that forms amyloid plaques. In a recent experiment on mice that were genetically defective so that they would develop amyloid deposits, scientists claimed success in immunizing the mice against overproduction of the harmful amyloid substance, thus preventing the production of amyloid deposits. This raises the very real prospect of the development of a human vaccine against AD. It is important to keep in mind, however, that both the APP and the presenilin genes, which have been linked to early-onset AD, account for only a small number of AD cases. Early-onset AD (which strikes before age 65, and has a clear genetic basis) is uncommon. In most cases, signs of AD appear only after age 65, with the risk rising with increased age. The more common late-onset AD has a much weaker genetic basis than early-onset AD.

One gene that does appear to play a role in some instances of late-onset AD produces a protein called *apolipoprotein E* (ApoE), believed by some researchers to play a critical role in maintaining the supply of vital nutrients to brain cells. The ApoE protein has three variants, each of which produces a slightly different version of the protein.

Every person inherits a variant of the ApoE gene from each parent, with the result that there are many possible combinations. Research at Duke University has determined that one of the variants, known as e4, confers a high risk for developing AD, especially if it is inherited from both parents. In fact, in this Duke University study, 91 percent of people who inherited e4 from both parents developed AD.

Again, though, genetics is only part of the story with late-onset AD. For one thing, the risk of developing late-onset AD is only slightly higher if one's parents, brothers, or sisters had, or has, AD. Also, only 3 percent of the population inherits the e4 variant of the ApoE gene from both parents. More than half the population, in fact, has the desirable e3/e3 combination. And finally, lacking the e4 variant of the gene does not guarantee one will not get AD. The same researchers determined that just 64 percent of AD patients without a family history of the disease had one or more e4 alleles.

AD has many causes

AD experts agree that AD, like dementia in general, is not a single disease with a single cause. Certain genes may predispose some people to AD, but not everyone, and others may develop AD without that genetic risk. Many lifestyle factors may play a role in turning a genetic AD risk into reality, and destructive habits of thought and behavior can in themselves be sufficient to cause impaired cognition and perhaps even dementia.

So much press is given to AD disease these days that we are all being distracted from some very important facts: There are many possible causes of apparent cognitive decline in adulthood and old age, and many of those causes respond readily to fairly low-tech treatment. Sometimes the treatment is as simple as making sure that you have enough social contact, mental stimulation, and physical exercise to keep your brain healthy. And while we are all waiting for an AD cure, we should not forget that many of the same factors that are bad for our brain at age 30 or 40 may also contribute to developing AD later in life. Finally, as more and more drugs and medications are developed to help reduce the risk of AD or to slow the progression of the disease once it starts, it is essential to keep in mind that those medications work better if they are accompanied by the things that have the power to help maintain a healthy brain in the first place.

DSM-IV Diagnostic Criteria For AD

The standard diagnostic manual for mental disorders, the DSM-IV, cites the following criteria for dementia of the Alzheimer's type:

A. Development of multiple cognitive deficits:

  (1) memory impairment (learning new information or recalling previously learned information), and

  (2) one or more of the following:

    (a) language disturbance

    (b) difficulty carrying out motor activities (such as using a can opener, making the bed)

    (c) difficulty identifying objects

    (d) executive function difficulties (planning, organizing, abstracting).

B. The deficits in (A) cause impairment in work or social settings and represent a decline from a previous level.

C. The deficits begin gradually and continue to get worse.

D. The deficits are not due to other causes, such as stroke, brain tumor, Parkinson's, hypothyroidism, vitamin deficiency, HIV, prescription or over-the-counter drugs, or alcohol.

E. The deficits do not only occur during delirium.

F. The deficits are not better accounted for by another mental disorder, such as depression or schizophrenia.

(Source: American Psychiatric Association (1994). *Diagnostic and Statistical Manual of Mental Disorders: DSM-IV.* Washington, D.C.: American Psychiatric Association.)

A Quick Screening Exam:
The Time and Change Test

This is a recently developed screening test for Alzheimer's and other dementias, created by researchers Froehlich, Robison, and Inouye. It has been shown to be very reliable in ruling out possible dementia, although very mild cases might still slip through.

TIME:
What time is it?
(Two tries allowed, maximum 1 minute.)

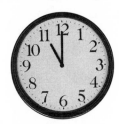

CHANGE:
   Select any coins that will add up to exactly one dollar. (2 tries allowed, maximum 2 minutes.)

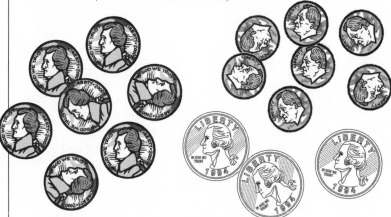

Scoring: If either question cannot be answered correctly, there is possible dementia. If both questions are answered correctly, dementia is less likely.

(Source: T.F. Froehlich, J.T. Robison, and S.K. Inouye (1998). Screening for dementia in the outpatient setting: the Time and Change Test. *Journal of the American Geriatric Society* 46:1506-11.)

A Short Mental Status Test

If you are worried about dementia, one of the first things to do is to get your physician, or a specialist recommended by your physician, to give you a preliminary mental status exam. This one is based on the Mini-Mental State Examination, designed by psychiatrists Folstein, Folstein, and McHugh in 1975, and still the most widely used preliminary screening test for dementia. This test is best done with two people, one to ask the questions and record the answers or point total. There is no time limit.

	Max Score	Score
		ORIENTATION
1)	5	What is the (1) date (2) year (3) day (4) month (5) season? (1 pt. each)
2)	5	Where are we? (If done at home) (1) state (2) county (3) town (4) street (5) house number (Adjust number 5 if not done at home.) (1 pt. each)
		REGISTRATION
3)	3	Examiner: Name three unrelated objects (e.g., chair, spoon, candlestick). Then, ask examinee to repeat them. (1 pt. for each object correctly repeated)
		ATTENTION AND CALCULATION
4)	5	Count backwards by sevens from 100 (93, 86, etc.). Stop after five answers. Or: Spell "world" backwards. (1 pt. each number or letter correct)
		RECALL
5)	3	What were the three objects mentioned in Question 3? (1 pt. each)

6)	2	LANGUAGE Examiner: Point to a pencil and a watch, and ask the examinee to name them. (1 pt. each)
7)	1	Repeat: "There's no such thing as a free lunch." (1 pt.)
8)	3	Follow this command: "Take a piece of paper, fold it in half, and put it on the floor." (1 pt. for each step)
9)	3	Read and follow these requests: (1) Point to your left ear (2) Write a sentence (3) Copy this design: (1 pt. each)

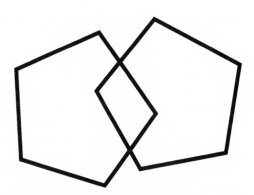

Scoring: A score of less than 25 means that cognitive impairment is likely — although not necessarily due to Alzheimer's — and that you should pursue further tests.

(Source: M.F. Folstein, S.E. Folstein, and P.R. McHugh (1975). Mini-mental state. *Journal of Psychiatric Research* 12: 189-98.)

Another Quick Screening Exam: The Set Test

This simple test for dementia, many variations of which are in use, was developed by psychiatrists Isaacs and Kennie in the early seventies. Like the Time and Change Test, it is very quick to take and easy to score.

For each of the following categories, allow 30 seconds to name as many items as you can (up to ten items per category):

      (1) colors   (2) animals

      (3) fruits   (4) towns

Scoring: 1 pt. for each correct item, for a maximum of 40 pts. total.
Less than 15: likely dementia, 15-24: possible dementia, 25+: no dementia

(Source: B. Isaacs and A.T. Kennie (1973). The Set Test as an aid to the detection of dementia in old people. *British Journal of Psychiatry* 123: 467-70.)

A Clinical Diagnosis of Probable AD Includes:

(1) Dementia established by a clinical exam and a mental status test such as the Mini-Mental State, and confirmed by neuropsychological tests;

(2) Deficits in at least two areas of cognition;

(3) Progressive worsening of memory and other cognitive abilities;

(4) No disturbance of consciousness;

(5) Onset between 40 and 90, usually after age 65;

(6) Absence of other disorders that could explain the dementia.

(Source: American Psychiatric Association (1994). *Diagnostic and Statistical Manual of Mental Disorders: DSM-IV.* Washington, D.C.: American Psychiatric Association.)

SOLUTIONS

The toothed plates numbered 2 and 4 will move toward each other and touch.

RUBE MONKEYBERG P. 136

a. 6, b. 27, c. None will have designs on four sides. Eight have designs on three sides. Twelve have designs on two sides. Six have designs on one side, d. 1

CUBE CUTUP P. 137

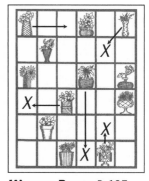

WINDOW BOXES P. 137

1. C
2. 2 and 4
3. 1
4. 5

BLOCK PARTY P. 139

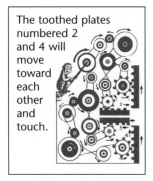

MATCH PATCH P. 140

A. Twenty-four stacks of white tiles for the center area. Nine stacks of white tiles for around the edge.

B. Twenty-three stacks of black tiles for the center area. Seven stacks of black tiles around the edge.

STACK ROOM P. 141

Carolyn sees two striped hats, Allen's and Wally's. She reasons that if her hat is striped, Allen and Wally will also see two striped hats, and their hands will stay up. Conversely, she reasons, if her hat is not striped, Allen and Wally will each see one striped hat (the other guy's) and one unstriped hat (hers). If this were the case, Allen would have raised his hand for Wally's striped hat, and vice versa, and because they're both pretty bright, it shouldn't take one of them long to figure out that he's the one wearing the striped hat the other guy is raising his hand for. Carolyn allows enough time for Allen or Wally to figure this out. Since neither does, Carolyn knows she must be wearing a striped hat too, and she lowers her hand.

PARTY HATS P. 142

No answer

MIND'S EYE P. 143

1. Bob
2. Tony
3. Dick
4. Harry
5. Tom

HAIRY PROBLEM P. 144

John likes math and lives in house A. Ed studies English. Lucy is into physics. Tina studies philosophy and Sir Rodney is her houseguest.

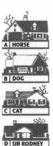

A HORSE

B DOG

C CAT

D SIR RODNEY

HOUSE GUEST P. 145

The girl wearing Daryl's dress and Karen's hat can't be Daryl or Karen so it must be Allyson. If Daryl is wearing Allyson's dress, Karen must be wearing her own. And since we know she is not, Daryl is wearing Karen's dress and Karen is wearing Allyson's

DRESS-UP TIME P. 146

The number in parenthesis indicates the clue reference.

Angie Pappas and Lorraine Dickinson showed roses. Bobbi Fellows exhibited pansies. Karen Kennedy displayed white carnations.

Angie didn't grow pansies (5), and since she was down three tables from Lorraine's she can't be the exhibitor of the white carnations. She must be a rose displayer. Lorraine didn't show white carnations (1), and neither did Bobbi (4), so the carnation displayer must be Karen. Lorraine didn't exhibit pansies (5), so she must have been the other woman who displayed roses. Bobby had the pansy arrangement. Karen's last name is not Pappas (2) or Fellows (6). Since she displayed carnations, her last name is not Dickinson (4) nor is Angie's (7), so Lorraine must be Mrs. Dickinson. Since Angie and Lorraine Dickinson displayed roses, Angie's last name isn't Fellows (3). Hers is Pappas and Bobbi's last name is Fellows.

FLOWER SHOW P. 147

---

1. From top to bottom: queen of clubs, ace of diamonds, ace of hearts, queen of diamonds.

2. From left to right: seven of hearts, king of spades, four of diamonds.

CARD SENSE P. 148

Pick up just one glass by *pouring* the wine from glass 5 into glass 2.

VIN ORDINAIRE P. 149

Here is one answer. Is yours as logical? Football-Pig (pigskin), Cat-Mouse, Dog-Hydrant, Bird-Birdhouse, Baseball-Cap, Cheese-Mousetrap, Bulb-Sun, Car-Rocket, Umbrella-Rubbers, Campfire-Tent.

PARTICULAR PAIRS P. 150

Left Brain Matches:
rain cloud — tornado
beach umbrella — sun
bugs — snail
top — noisy kids
igloo — house
bowler hat — beanie
crying lady — happy man

Right Brain Matches:
rain cloud — crying lady
beach umbrella — beanie
top — tornado
igloo — bowler hat
sun — happy man
bugs — noisy kids
snail — house

POSSIBLE PAIRS P. 151

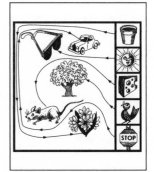

TANGLE TRACE P. 152

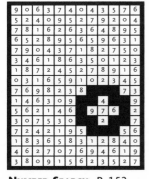

NUMBER SEARCH P. 153

The silhouette in box 6 and the picture in box 7 exactly match the picture in box 1. Silhouette 2 is missing the foot on the bowl. Picture 3 is missing a small flower on the right. Silhouette 4 is missing leaves on the center thistle. Picture 5 is missing the stem of the tulip in the center. Silhouette 8 is missing a small cluster on the right. Picture 9 is missing a dotted stalk on the left.

FLOWER DISARRANGEMENT P. 154

From top to bottom:
D-2, B-3,
B-8, A-2, E-1,
B-6, E-9.

MATCH BOXES P. 155

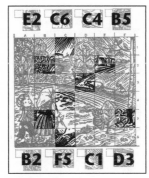

MISSING PIECES P. 156

A-7, B-5, C-3, D-9, E-1, F-6, G-2, H-8, J-4

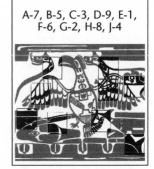

MENTAL JIGSAW P. 157

187

The symbols, when translated into numbers, are arranged in this sequential grouping: (1), (1, 2), (1, 2, 3), (1, 2, 3, 4), (1, 2, 3, 4, 5), (1, 2, 3, 4, 5, 6), (1, 2, 3, 4, 5, 6, 7), (1, 2, 3, 4, 5, 6, 7, 8). The answer is the triangle, symbol 3.

PLAY THE SYMBOLS P. 158

B6, C1 or C2, E2 or E4, E5.

TANGRAM P. 159

Pronouncing "PH" as in "prophet" = "F"; "WR" as in "wreck" = "R"; "EG" as in "phlegm" = "E"; "T" as in "position" = "SH"; "GH" as in "cough" = "F"; "O" as in "women" = "I"; "SS" as in "issue" = "SH." Or: FRESH FISH.

PHUNNEY PHONETICS P. 160

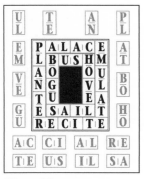

WORD MIX-UP P. 161

NEGOTIATION
REBATED
TRANSLATE
ARCHDUCHESS
STRUGGLING
TRESPASSERS
PROMOTE
CONDUCTOR
_ _ _EVINCE_ _ _
FOLLOW EVINCE ✓
DADDY ROTATE

LETTER LOGIC P. 162

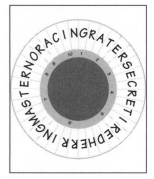

TWISTS & TURNS P. 163

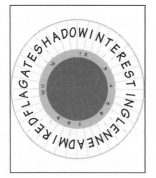

BRRRRR! P. 164

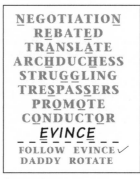

IS				WORD	
IS		COOL	WOOD	WOOD	
SKIRT		COOT	WOOL	WOOL	
SHIRT	BOOT	FOOL			
SHORT	BOUT	FOUL			
SHORE	POUT	SOUL			
WHORE	POUR	SOUR			
WHERE	YOUR	YOUR			

	BOILS	LOPES	
DIE	TOILS	LOBES	
DOE	TOOLS	ROBES	
ROE	TOOTS	ROSES	
ROW	TOOTH	POSES	
POW	SOOTH	POSEY	
POT	MOUTH	MOSEY	
PUT	MOUTH	MONEY	

LADDERGRAM/CHANGEUPS P. 165

WORD SPIRAL P. 166

188

G5 CUBA	C4 BORNEO
C7 LAOS	H1 CYPRUS
F1 OMAN	D7 ISRAEL
G3 PERU	C2 GAMBIA
	C2 GUINEA
C4 BURMA	A4 NORWAY
A7 INDIA	E6 BRAZIL
E4 ITALY	
C7 LIBYA	H8 ALGERIA
G3 PANAMA	F3 AUSTRIA
D6 SYRIA	C4 BRITAIN
F8 ZAIRE	C2 GERMANY
	B1 LEBANON
H5 BULGARIA	C7 LIBERIA
	H7 NIGERIA
	E2 ROMANIA

WORDS ANY-WAY P. 168

5 items at $25	=	$125
4 items at $3	=	12
3 items at $1	=	3
2 items at $50	=	100
1 item at $20	=	20
Total		$260

ANTIQUE ACCOUNTING P. 169

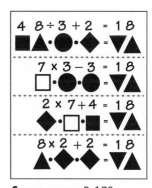

SYMBOLATICS P. 170

A. Square the difference between the first and second numbers. Thus the difference between 17 and 11 is six, squared equals 36.

B. C is double the total of A plus B. E is double the total of C plus D. G. which is double the total of E plus F, equals 104.

12	4	64
9	6	9
17	11	36

A	B	C	D	E	F	G
2	4	12	8	40	12	**104**

MISSING DIGITS P. 171

1. $11 \times 4 = 22 \times 2$
2. $9 / 3 = 9 - 6$
3. $10 + 8 = 18$
4. $77 / 11 = 7$
5. $3 \times 6 = 18$
6. $8 + 1 = 9$
7. $5 + 3 = 8$

MATCH STICKLERS P. 172

189

Index